100 Questions & Answers About Macular Degeneration

Jeffrey S. Heier, MD
Ophthalmic Consultants of Boston
Assistant Professor of Ophthalmology,
Tufts School of Medicine
Clinical Instructor of Ophthalmology,
Harvard Medical School
Boston, Massachusetts

JONES

BOSTON

World Headquarters
Jones and Bartlett Publishers
40 Tall Pine Drive
Sudbury, MA 01776
978-443-5000
info@jbpub.com
www.jbpub.com

Jones and Bartlett Publishers
Canada
6339 Ormindale Way
Mississauga, Ontario L5V 1J2
Canada

Jones and Bartlett Publishers
International
Barb House, Barb Mews
London W6 7PA
United Kingdom

Jones and Bartlett's books and products are available through most bookstores and online book-sellers. To contact Jones and Bartlett Publishers directly, call 800-832-0034, fax 978-443-8000, or visit our website, www.jbpub.com.

Substantial discounts on bulk quantities of Jones and Bartlett's publications are available to corporations, professional associations, and other qualified organizations. For details and specific discount information, contact the special sales department at Jones and Bartlett via the above contact information or send an email to specialsales@jbpub.com.

The authors, editor, and publisher have made every effort to provide accurate information. However, they are not responsible for errors, omissions, or for any outcomes related to the use of the contents of this book and take no responsibility for the use of the products and procedures described. Treatments and side effects described in this book may not be applicable to all people; likewise, some people may require a dose or experience a side effect that is not described herein. Drugs and medical devices are discussed that may have limited availability controlled by the Food and Drug Administration (FDA) for use only in a research study or clinical trial. Research, clinical practice, and government regulations often change the accepted standard in this field. When consideration is being given to use of any drug in the clinical setting, the healthcare provider or reader is responsible for determining FDA status of the drug, reading the package insert, and reviewing prescribing information for the most up-to-date recommendations on dose, precautions, and contraindications, and determining the appropriate usage for the product. This is especially important in the case of drugs that are new or seldom used.

Production Credits
Executive Publisher: Chris Davis
Editorial Assistant: Sara Cameron
Production Director: Amy Rose
Associate Production Editor: Jessica deMartin
Photo Researcher: Carolyn Arcabascio
Manufacturing and Inventory Control Supervisor: Amy Bacus
Composition: Glyph International
Printing and Binding: Malloy, Inc.

Cover Credits
Cover Design: Carolyn Downer
Cover Printing: Malloy, Inc.
Cover Images: Top left: T-Design/Shutterstock, Inc.; Top right: Absolut/Shutterstock, Inc.; Bottom: Andresr/Shutterstock, Inc.

Library of Congress Cataloging-in-Publication Data
Heier, Jeffrey S.
    100 questions & answers about macular degeneration / Jeffrey Heier.—1st ed.
        p. cm.
    Includes index.
    ISBN 978-0-7637-6436-4 (alk. paper)
1. Retinal degeneration—Miscelleana. 2. Retinal degeneration—Popular works. I. Title.
II. Title: One hundred questions and answers about macular degeneration.
    RE661.D3H47 2010
    617.7' 35—dc22
                                                                                2009038490
6048

Printed in the United States of America
13 12 11 10 09   10 9 8 7 6 5 4 3 2 1

This book is dedicated to my daughters, Brittany and Alexandra, whose beauty, grace, and love are the light of my life; and to my beautiful wife, Polly, without whose love, support, and understanding my work would not be possible.

Contents

Questions 1–16 discuss the basics of macular degeneration, including:
- What is age-related macular degeneration (AMD)?
- Will I go blind from macular degeneration?
- What is a low vision specialist, and how can he or she help me?

Questions 17–25 review the different variables that can lead to macular degeneration, such as:
- What are the risk factors for age-related macular degeneration?
- Are men or women more likely to get age-related macular degeneration?
- I have a family history of macular degeneration. Is there anything I can do to avoid getting it myself?

Questions 26–38 explain the components of dry age-related macular degeneration:
- How is dry macular degeneration diagnosed?
- What are the early symptoms of dry macular degeneration?
- I understand that new medicines are available to treat wet macular degeneration. Will these medicines also help my dry macular degeneration?

Questions 39–48 describe numerous ways you can help control your macular degeneration through diet and vitamins, including:
- Are vitamin supplements recommended for all patients with age-related macular degeneration? Even if they aren't recommended for my stage of macular degeneration, will it hurt me to take them?

Some Introductory Questions and Answers

How does it feel to find out that you or someone close to you has age-related macular degeneration (AMD)?

Frightening.

What can help to combat that fear?

It helps to understand AMD—the disease process, its risk factors, how it is treated, what the prognosis for that treatment is, how it will impact your life, and what can be done to cope. Taking ownership of understanding what is going on with your eyes or your loved one's eyes is a way of getting back some control. One way to take ownership is to ask questions.

Is AMD a confusing disease?

Yes, it is. Even the name "age-related macular degeneration" is confusing; literally it just means that something is wrong with the center part of the retina, and it gets worse as you age. Moreover, AMD has many different forms, new information about it is available almost daily, many new studies are being performed, and treatment recommendations continue to change—a recipe for confusion.

What other things make AMD a challenge?

Visual loss strikes at the very heart of the human condition. Our independence, our joys in life, and our sense of self are intimately wrapped up in our visual perception of the world and our ability to navigate in it. AMD threatens all of this.

Who is best at answering questions about AMD?

Retina specialists who have many years of experience treating AMD and explaining it to patients are particularly effective at answering questions. Dr. Heier is not only one of the top AMD experts in the world, he is also a superb and compassionate communicator.

What questions should I ask?

This book can help. Dr. Heier and his team have picked the questions they are asked the most. And they have answered them clearly and concisely. There is a lot of information here. This book is a superb place for you to start.

You are fortunately entering the AMD arena at a time when our knowledge is expanding exponentially and, along with it, our treatment options. The prognosis for vision has improved dramatically for AMD patients just in the last few years, and there is every reason to believe that it will continue to do so.

The diagnosis of AMD is one of the big challenges that life can put before us. With good medical care, that challenge can be met and conquered. This book is an essential guide to navigating that challenging path. Good luck and safe travels!

Julia A. Haller, MD
Ophthalmologist-in-Chief
Wills Eye Institute
Professor and Chair of Ophthalmology
Jefferson Medical College
Thomas Jefferson University

Over the last several years, we have seen dramatic advances in the diagnosis and treatment of age-related macular degeneration (AMD). These advances have largely addressed wet macular degeneration, the form that is the least common overall (dry macular degeneration is far more common), but by far the most common cause of severe vision loss secondary to dry AMD. I first began caring for patients with this devastating disease almost 20 years ago as an ophthalmologist in training. In those days, the diagnosis of wet AMD was met with extreme frustration and disappointment, as there were no effective therapies that helped to improve vision and few that even helped to stabilize it. The diagnosis, if involving the fellow eye of a patient who already had wet disease in one eye, often meant a loss of independence for the patient and possible, if not probable, commitment to an assisted living environment or significant burden to a family support system.

From 2000 to 2004, several advances in the treatment of wet AMD significantly improved our ability to help these patients, including a type of cold laser and an intraocular injection (Macugen). However, despite each of these treatments representing an improvement to our then current approach, they each still had one major drawback—while each of these treatments was effective at slowing visual loss, neither resulted in an overall improvement in vision. In other words, if offered one of these treatments, the patient was still likely to lose vision, but the loss may not have been as extensive or as quick as if they were offered no treatment at all. Hardly an encouraging prospect for already upset patients.

Everything changed in the summer of 2005. The study results of a new drug, Lucentis, were reported, and for the first time a treatment actually stopped progression in the large majority of patients with wet AMD. Even more exciting, a significant percentage (30–40%) actually gained several lines of vision (as measured on an eye chart). This represented a dramatic improvement over any treatments seen up to that time. Over the same summer, clinicians began to use another drug, Avastin, which was approved as a cancer therapy a year earlier but had similar characteristics to Lucentis. This use was off-label (meaning it was being used for an indication for which it had not been approved) and, therefore, not as well studied as Lucentis, but the drug was also demonstrating promising results. Finally, hope for wet AMD patients was not only on the horizon, it had exploded upon us. No longer is the diagnosis of wet AMD an ocular death sentence; it has become a very treatable disease that has a high likelihood of being halted and a reasonable chance of visual recovery.

As success with wet AMD has been achieved, clinicians and researchers have recognized that dry AMD is another problem altogether. Now that wet disease is treated effectively, substantial efforts are being directed to the damaging effects of dry disease. And these efforts are reaping benefits. Exciting discoveries into previously unknown mechanisms of disease progression, coupled with revolutionary breakthroughs regarding genetic aspects of both wet and dry disease, are leading the way. Potential innovative approaches to dry disease, as well as new therapies for wet disease, are in the lab and clinical trials even as this book is being written. It is likely that additional advances are in our future. Being diagnosed with age-related macular degeneration is never a good thing, but the prognosis for maintaining useful vision is so much greater today than it was even a few years ago. And the prognosis a few years from now will likely be even better.

This book was written to help alleviate the fear of this all-too-common disease. Had I been asked to write this book 10 years ago, or even 5, I would have declined, as I would have felt that it couldn't convey the hope or promise that I would have desired. Fortunately, the advances over the last several years make this book not only reasonable, but necessary. Patients and their families need to better understand AMD. Questions such as what is it, how can it be recognized, is it preventable, and how is it treated are common, but they are frequently asked and answered in the office environment where time and circumstances aren't ideal for understanding. This book allows patients and their families an opportunity to organize their thoughts and questions and to digest the answers in the comfort and calm of their own home. These questions are based on years of experience taking care of thousands of AMD patients and their families, and they were compiled with the help of my outstanding research staff who, like myself, care for these patients daily. This book is not intended to replace the critical interactions and discussions between patients and their retina specialists, but we hope it will enable patients to better understand their disease and the future. Numerous patients with AMD have asked each and every one of these questions, and the answers are those that helped them to better understand their disease and to approach it in a knowledgeable, positive manner.

Jeffrey S. Heier, MD

I had retired from a chaotic 30-year career in real estate and was pursuing something that I really loved, when my world collapsed around me.

I had attended a woodworking class, which led a waterfowl carving class. I really loved the carving and was chasing it by taking courses, traveling to shows, and having personal instruction. I lived in Cape Ann, Massachusetts, and the inspiration abounded for waterfowl carving. I had found my niche.

One day, while looking at clapboards of a neighborhood house, I noted that the lines were all wavy, rather than horizontal and straight. Having been told emphatically that I should notify my glaucoma doctor if I noticed any changes in my sight, I went to him immediately.

He examined me and asked if I could immediately see Dr. Jeffrey S. Heier, to whom he would refer me. I was a little shocked but said of course. I went that same day to see Dr. Heier in Boston. And thus began my journey with AMD. My dry macular degeneration had turned wet, and my vision was going. I was expecting the worst. Instead, I was fortunate to get into a trial of the drug that became Lucentis. When Dr. Heier diagnosed me with wet AMD in my left eye, my vision in that eye was measured at 20/200. Only 3 months before, my vision had been 20/30 in that eye, so the loss of vision happened quickly. Dr. Heier enrolled me in the clinical trial, and I began receiving the study treatment, Lucentis.

My vision steadily improved with this treatment, and I was thrilled. Unfortunately, about a year and a half after being diagnosed with wet AMD in my left eye, my right eye developed it. At that time

(2003), Lucentis was only being tested in clinical trials, and there was no way to receive the treatment in my second eye, even though my study eye had responded well. The vision in my right eye continued to deteriorate despite receiving treatments clinically available at that time, and today it measures at 20/400. Thankfully, being treated in my left eye with Lucentis was very successful for me, and I regained my total vision in that eye.

Today I enjoy a very happy and full life, carving, skiing, boating, and reading. I am so grateful for the opportunity I was given.

Nicholas Fairfield

Acknowledgments

The critically important job of caring for patients and undertaking macular degeneration research would not be possible without the amazing clinical and research staff with whom I am fortunate to work every day at Ophthalmic Consultants of Boston. I have had the privilege of working with many talented individuals in the past and present, and my patients and I are eternally grateful. Several of them helped to select the questions answered in this book. They are Sandy Chong, Leah Cox, and Robin Ty. One individual in particular, Alison Nowak, has helped with this project from start to finish, and while it would have been completed without her help, it would have taken at least twice as long.

I would also like to thank Dr. Chirag Shah and Dr. Grant Janzen for reviewing the completed manuscript and providing their valuable and poignant insight.

Finally, I would like to thank Nicholas Fairfield, the extraordinary sculptor, who developed macular degeneration and continued to produce remarkable pieces of work despite impaired vision in one eye. His comments add tremendous insight to many questions in this book.

PART ONE

Background: What Is It, Where Is It, and Who Has It?

What is age-related macular degeneration (AMD)?

Will I go blind from macular degeneration?

What is a low vision specialist, and how can he or she help me?

More . . .

1. What is age-related macular degeneration (AMD)?

Age-related **macular degeneration** is a degenerative disease affecting the center part of the retina known as the **macula**. The macula, which is described in more detail in Question 3, is the center part of the retina that is responsible for central vision. Central vision is what is used to perform activities requiring visual detail such as reading, recognizing faces, or driving a car. Macular degeneration is the leading cause of visual loss in patients over 50 years of age in the United States.

Age-related macular degeneration is often classified as one of two types. The first type, known as **dry macular degeneration**, involves gradual breakdown of the macula. It is characterized by certain findings, including **drusen**, which are yellow-white spots in the macula and outside of the macula, as well as degenerative changes in several layers of the macula. These changes may involve **atrophy** (loss of tissue) or **hyperpigmentation** (clumping of pigment cells). These changes may be mild and may result in few or no symptoms. With advanced disease, these changes may become more prevalent and may result in mild, moderate, or significant visual loss. In the most advanced stages of dry macular degeneration, you can actually experience complete loss of critical layers of the retina, known as **geographic atrophy**. When geographic atrophy involves the center of the macula, it results in severe visual loss. Fortunately, geographic atrophy occurs in only a minority of patients.

Wet macular degeneration occurs when an abnormal growth of blood vessels underneath or into the macula results in leakage or bleeding. As you would imagine, leakage or bleeding in the retina often leads to significant visual symptoms and can result in sudden and dramatic loss of central vision.

Macular degeneration

The breakdown over time of the cells in the macula. Macular degeneration can occur from a number of causes, one of which is aging, and is referred to as age-related macular degeneration.

Macula

The central area of the retina that is critical for fine, detailed vision.

Dry macular degeneration

The deterioration of the layers of the retina secondary to abnormal aging changes in the eye. This is the most common form of macular degeneration.

Drusen

Yellow deposits beneath the retina, often indicative of macular degeneration. Drusen can be small and hard, large and soft, or anywhere in between.

Atrophy

A progressive breakdown or wasting away of a tissue, such as that seen in advanced dry macular degeneration.

At this time, vitamin supplementation offers the only approved treatment for dry macular degeneration, and it is geared toward preventing or slowing progression of disease. Fortunately, significant advances have occurred in the treatment of wet macular degeneration, as will be discussed in depth later in the book. It should be noted that all cases of wet macular degeneration originate from dry macular degeneration; however, the majority of patients who have dry macular degeneration will not progress to wet disease. Approximately 10% of patients with dry macular degeneration will develop the wet form of the disease.

2. What is the retina?

The **retina** (**Figure 1**) is the tissue lining the inside of the eye. It is a light-sensitive tissue that lines most of the eye, excluding the clear front part of the eye (the cornea). It is easiest to think of the eye as a camera. The **cornea** is the clear part or the lens of the camera, and the retina is the film. Images enter through the clear part of the eye and when they strike the retina, they stimulate impulses, which are transmitted through the **optic nerve** to the brain. The brain then interprets these impulses into images. If the film in a camera is bad or damaged, the images are not clear.

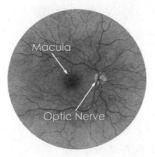

Figure 1   The Retina.

Background

Hyperpigmentation

Increased pigmentation (black or dark coloring) at the level of the retina. Hyperpigmentation indicates increased risk of macular degeneration progressing.

Geographic atrophy (GA)

Geographic atrophy is the advanced form of dry macular degeneration in which critical layers of the retina break down or degenerate entirely. When GA involves the center of the macula, severe vision loss may occur.

Wet macular degeneration

Damage and breakdown of the retina in which an abnormal growth of new blood vessels results in leakage and bleeding beneath and into the retina.

Retina

The tissue lining the inner surface of the eye that receives light impulses and transmits them through the optic nerve to the brain.

Cornea

The clear, dome-shaped front part of the eye. The cornea helps to focus light onto the retina.

Optic nerve

The nerve that transmits impulses from the retina to the brain.

Similarly, if the retina is damaged, as in macular degeneration, the images are not clear.

3. What is the macula?

The macula (**Figure 2**) is the center part of the retina responsible for clear central vision. The macula actually occupies only a small part of the overall retina but is critically important to vision. It is the macula that is capable of reading, recognizing faces, driving, etc. The macula is also the part of the retina that allows one to see color. Diseases that damage the entire retina but spare the macula may be associated with 20/20 vision (although it will appear as tunnel vision). Such diseases include **retinitis pigmentosa** and **glaucoma**. On the other hand, diseases or injuries that affect the macula but spare the rest of the retina are associated with terrible central vision, often 20/200 or worse, even though the peripheral vision is unaffected.

Retinitis pigmentosa (RP)

A group of inherited retinal disorders characterized by progressive visual field loss and difficulty with night vision.

Glaucoma

A group of diseases that cause optic nerve damage and visual field loss as a result of intraocular pressure that is too high for the health of the eye. In some patients, this pressure is much higher than normal, but in others, even intraocular pressure that falls within the normal range may not be tolerated by an eye (so-called low-tension glaucoma). Glaucoma is typically treated with either eye drops or surgery (either intraocular or laser), or a combination of both.

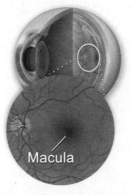

Figure 2　The Macula.

4. How many people have age-related macular degeneration in the United States?

The presence of some degree of age-related macular degeneration in elderly patients in the United States is quite common. Somewhere between 10 and 15 million elderly Americans have some form of age-related macular degeneration. Seven million Americans are believed to be at high risk of developing wet macular degeneration from their dry form due to the presence of large drusen. Large drusen are a known risk factor for progression to the wet form of macular degeneration.

Advanced age-related macular degeneration affects 1.75 million Americans. Advanced age-related macular degeneration includes wet macular degeneration and geographic atrophy, the dry form of macular degeneration that can result in significant visual loss. The majority of patients with advanced macular degeneration have wet disease. It is estimated that 200,000 patients develop new wet macular degeneration annually.

With numbers such as these, it is obvious why so much time, effort, and financial resources are devoted to research of age-related macular degeneration. The U.S. aging population is growing, and it is estimated that the number of patients with advanced macular degeneration will increase to nearly 3 million Americans by the year 2020.

5. Is age-related macular degeneration truly age related? If so, at what age should we be concerned?

The risk of age-related macular degeneration and subsequent visual loss clearly increases with age. The risk of visual loss in patients under 50 years of age is uncommon. From 50 to 60 years of age, it is unlikely, but data show that the risk increases significantly in those 60 years and older. The risk in people 50 years of age or younger of developing any type of macular

Somewhere between 10 and 15 million elderly Americans have some form of age-related macular degeneration.

Background

degeneration is 2%, but this risk increases to nearly 30% in those 75 years or older.

6. Can a younger person have macular degeneration?

Yes, although questions remain as to whether this is truly age-related macular degeneration or simply another form of macular degeneration. Younger patients can develop drusen and pigment changes characteristic of those seen in older patients with the diagnosis of age-related macular degeneration. Debate exists as to whether or not this is the same disease as age-related macular degeneration or a different disease entirely. These macular changes would still be termed macular degeneration, as it does involve a degeneration of the macula; however, when seen in younger patients, it obviously is not age-related. The appearance of drusen in younger patients has been termed familial or hereditary drusen, but their absolute risk of progression to advanced stages of macular degeneration is not yet known. Other variants of macular degeneration may exist in younger patients and merit careful evaluation and follow-up by an ophthalmologist.

7. What is a cataract, and how can I tell the difference between macular degeneration and my cataract?

Cataract

A clouding of one's natural lens.

A **cataract** is a clouding of the natural lens of the eye. The lens of the eye helps to focus, or direct, images from the front of the eye onto the retina. It must be clear and free of opacities or abnormalities in order to focus the images clearly on the retina. The retina then takes these images and transmits signals to the brain. Some of the symptoms of macular degeneration and cataracts overlap. Blurred vision can be due to either problem; however, age-related macular degeneration is more likely to cause distorted or wavy vision. Cataracts, on the other hand, are more likely to cause problems with glare and significant blurring or double vision. Glare can be recognized when driving at night (you may have increased difficulty ignoring oncoming headlights) or even during the day with bright sunlight. While all of us are sensitive to varying degrees of bright lights, cataracts result in a scattering of the light, which makes it even more difficult to see. Double vision is also a symptom of cataracts, or of some form of opacity in front of the retina, but is not a symptom of problems with the retina and therefore not a symptom of macular degeneration.

8. Can cataract surgery affect my age-related macular degeneration?

This has been a somewhat controversial question, as many patients have both cataracts and age-related macular degeneration. As patients' cataracts have progressed, some have held off vision-improving surgery due to the fear of it impacting their macular degeneration. Studies have been conflicting in responding to this question; however, the most recent data from the **Age-Related Eye Disease Study (AREDS)** have dispelled the belief that cataract surgery increases the likelihood of developing wet macular degeneration. Therefore, the current recommendation is that patients should consider cataract surgery if their daily activities are affected by the symptoms of the cataract.

Sometimes it can be difficult to determine whether visual symptoms are related to the cataract or the age-related macular degeneration. Blurred and cloudy vision and glare are more likely related to cataracts, and distorted or absent vision is more likely related to the

Age-Related Eye Disease Study (AREDS)

A multicenter national trial sponsored by the National Eye Institute, a branch of the National Institutes of Health, that showed that high levels of antioxidants and zinc (in combination with cupric oxide) reduced the risk of advanced macular degeneration and vision loss associated with this disease.

macular degeneration. However, these symptoms are not absolute, and your retina specialist will be helpful in making this determination.

Nick's comment:

At the point of the "trial" period when Lucentis was clearly helping my left eye, my right eye developed wet macular degeneration. Unfortunately, since it was still an investigational drug, I could not get Lucentis for my right eye. Soon after this, a cataract was removed from my right eye. I was told to remove the bandage the afternoon following surgery, and I could not believe what I could see peripherally even though my central vision had deteriorated due to macular degeneration. This cataract operation helped my sight dramatically. I am very grateful.

9. Will I go blind from macular degeneration?

Total blindness from macular degeneration is extremely rare.

Visual field

The total area in which vision exists while staring straight ahead at a fixed point. This typically refers to peripheral vision.

No. Total blindness from macular degeneration is extremely rare. Macular degeneration typically affects the central part of vision, referred to as the macula. The macula actually represents a very small component of a patient's overall **visual field**. Therefore, while central vision can be significantly compromised, a patient's peripheral field (vision outside of the center) is not affected. This knowledge is reassuring to most patients with macular degeneration. Although central vision is extremely important for activities such as reading, watching television, and recognizing faces, peripheral vision is helpful for maintaining some degree of independence, walking, and avoiding bumping into things. Many patients confuse or mistake the idea of legal blindness with true blindness. These terms are addressed in the following question.

10. What is the difference between true blindness and legal blindness?

True blindness is when an eye is not capable of seeing any images or light. Even extremely bright lights directed right at the eye are not seen. **Legal blindness** refers to an eye's ability to read a certain level on a Snellen eye chart. The Snellen eye chart is the standard eye chart that is used at an eye care provider's office to measure and record vision. The large E on the Snellen eye chart refers to 20/400 vision, and the next line is recorded as 20/200 vision. Patients who are legally blind cannot read any further down on the eye chart than the 20/200 line. This means they may read the 20/200 line, the 20/400 line, or none of the eye chart. Legal blindness is determined by the best-seeing eye. For patients to be declared legally blind, neither of their eyes would be capable of reading better than 20/200. Patients who are unable to read better than 20/200 in one eye but capable of better vision in their fellow eye are not considered legally blind. For instance, if the bad eye is 20/400 and the good eye is 20/80, then the patient's best vision is considered 20/80, and he or she would not be considered legally blind. If legally blind, individuals may be eligible for certain benefits, including a possible deduction on income tax, as well as help from various businesses and organizations (such as unlimited directory assistance from the phone company or visual aids from state commissions for the blind).

True blindness

Also called total blindness, the complete lack of sight. Patients aren't even able to see light.

Legal blindness

Corrected vision (meaning with glasses if needed) that is 20/200 or worse in a patient's best-seeing eye.

Background

11. What is meant by a vision of 20/20 or 20/200?

Vision is measured by eye charts placed at standard distances from a patient. The Snellen eye chart is the standard eye chart used for measuring visual acuity in eye clinics as well as many physicians' offices. The first number, the 20, refers to the distance that the patient stands from the eye chart, conventionally 20 feet. The second number is the distance at which a person with normal, good vision would be standing to read the same letter that the patient reads from 20 feet. For instance, suppose a patient has terrible vision and is recorded at 20/200—this patient, while standing 20 feet from the eye chart, can read only at a level that a person with normal, good vision could read while standing 200 feet from the eye chart. Therefore, a patient with 20/20 vision has good vision and is able to see the same letters on the chart as a normal person at 20 feet.

Another example would be a patient who has 20/50 vision. This patient's vision is somewhat compromised, and when standing 20 feet from the eye chart, he or she can only read the same letters that a person with normal, good vision could read while standing 50 feet from the eye chart. Occasionally, patients have vision that is better than 20/20, and they might be recorded as 20/15. This means that when they stand 20 feet from the eye chart, a person with normal, good vision would actually have to move closer and stand 15 feet from the eye chart to see the same level. When individuals see better than 20/20, it means their vision is better than the normal standard for visual acuity.

Nick's comment:

I have one eye at 20/20 (the eye that received Lucentis) and one with no central vision. My peripheral vision in my poor eye is extremely important and a great help to me.

12. I have often heard macular degeneration referred to simply as "macula." Is macula another word for macular degeneration?

Macula is not an abbreviation for macular degeneration. While many people refer to macular degeneration simply as "macula," this is not accurate. The macula is the small critical area of the retina responsible for central vision. There are many diseases that affect the macula, including age-related macular degeneration, infectious diseases such as **histoplasmosis**, and hereditary diseases such as retinitis pigmentosa; therefore, referring to age-related macular degeneration as macula is not accurate.

Although the macula is actually a very small portion of the much larger retina, damage to it can result in severe vision loss. Damage outside of the macula, even if extensive, can have minimal effect on visual acuity because the central vision is spared. For instance, people can have retinal detachments with a significant portion of the retina detached, but if the macula is uninvolved, their vision is still often 20/20, although their visual field or peripheral vision is limited. Conversely, patients who have macular degeneration with involvement of only the very center of the retina may have significant visual loss, even to the point of 20/200 vision or worse, despite having perfect peripheral vision. These examples highlight the importance of the macula and underlie why our treatment of macular degeneration is so important.

13. What is a low vision specialist, and how can he or she help me?

A **low vision specialist** is someone who has been trained to maximize individuals' ability to utilize their impaired vision. Vision can be maximized through a

Histoplasmosis
A fungal infection that can occur in the retina. Its presence can lead to new blood vessel growth similar to that seen in wet macular degeneration.

Low vision specialist
A trained eye care provider (typically an optometrist or ophthalmologist) who evaluates and manages patients with impaired vision.

variety of methods. On one end of the spectrum, it may simply involve changing a patient's glasses prescription or increasing the magnification used for reading. More advanced intervention may be achieved with telescopic lenses that are clipped onto the outside of a spectacle correction. Monitors or devices that enlarge print, such as those in **Figure 3**, are also commonly used. In addition,

(a)

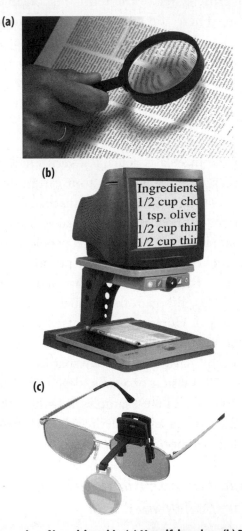

(b)

(c)

Figure 3   Examples of low vision aids. (a) Magnifying glass. (b) Desktop video magnifier. (c) Monocular magnifier clipped to eyeglasses.

(a) © Velychko/Shutterstock, Inc. (b) Courtesy of Freedom Scientific (c) Courtesy of Eschenbach Optik of America extensive training that may help a patient adapt to these techniques often proves invaluable in maximizing a patient's ability to perform daily activities.

Low vision help requires significant effort on both the patient's and the specialist's part; however, it can be extremely beneficial when properly applied. Low vision help is not meant to replace medical or surgical treatment of macular degeneration, nor is medical or surgical treatment exclusive of low vision help. They often work hand-in-hand to maximize patients' ability to get the most of their impaired or limited vision.

Low vision rehabilitation involves training in the utilization of low vision techniques as they apply to activities of daily living, such as cooking, performing a job, or getting around one's home or outside. Rehabilitation services typically involve a team of highly trained professionals (often led by an **ophthalmologist** or **optometrist**) who individualize the aforementioned aids to a person's unique situation.

Ophthalmologist
A medical doctor trained in the medical and surgical management of eye diseases.

Optometrist
A licensed healthcare professional trained to provide primary eye care.

14. How do I qualify for help from my state's Commission for the Blind?

State Commissions for the Blind provide a wide range of social and rehabilitation services to legally blind residents of all ages. Services are available based on an individual's needs and interests and are provided free of charge. Individuals can qualify for help from their state's Commission for the Blind if they meet the definition of legal blindness. This definition is dependent upon visual acuity being 20/200 or worse in the person's better-seeing eye, meaning that the person must be 20/200 or worse in both eyes. If one eye is 20/200 and the other slightly better, say 20/80 or 20/100, then the individual would not qualify for the definition of legal blindness and would not qualify for assistance from his or her state Commission for the Blind.

Some of the services include:

- Vocational rehabilitation services
- Social services
- Children's services
- Orientation and mobility services
- Deaf-blind services
- Rehabilitation teachers

Benefits include:

- Real estate tax exemptions
- Auto excise tax exemptions
- State and federal income tax exemptions/deductions
- Handicap parking placard or plates.

15. Are there online sources that can help me?

Yes. In the age of the Internet, the majority of organizations that provide information and/or support for macular degeneration patients also have Web sites. These organizations and their Web sites include, but are not limited to, the following:

- AMD Alliance International: www.amdalliance.org
- American Foundation for the Blind: www.afb.org
- American Macular Degeneration Foundation: www. macular.org
- Foundation Fighting Blindness: www.blindness.org
- National Eye Institute: www.nei.nih.gov/health/maculardegen
- Prevent Blindness America: www.preventblindness.org

Other, less specific sources such as Wikipedia (a free online encyclopedia) are very informative and can be extremely helpful (http://en.wikipedia.org/wiki/Macular_degeneration).

This list is by no means meant to be a complete or comprehensive listing of available Web sites. It is solely meant to serve as an initial aid in learning more on the Internet. Many of these sites offer an easy means of enlarging the print font for easier low-vision reading. One can access additional sites on the Web by performing a search—on Google, for instance—of "age-related macular degeneration," "macular degeneration," "ARMD," "or AMD." More specific questions, such as treatments or vitamin supplementation, may be easily searched as well.

16. Is there an association between macular degeneration and depression?

Many patients who develop macular degeneration also experience depression. The depression is a normal response to the fear of their current lifestyle being dramatically impacted. They are afraid they will experience a loss of independence, which a loss of vision might produce. Some patients already have depression, and macular degeneration simply worsens it. Others already have depression for which they are receiving treatment.

It is extremely important for patients who are experiencing depression to discuss this with their family members, with both their primary care physician and their retina specialist, and perhaps even with other patients or support groups. In many cases, a better understanding of the disease and the possible treatment options will help to alleviate some of the depression. In other cases, help with daily activities such as

In most cases, simply understanding the disease state and the help available can mitigate or eliminate depression.

that provided by low vision experts or the Commission for the Blind will also help to relieve the depression. In most cases, simply understanding the disease state and the help available can mitigate or eliminate depression.

Nick's comment:

I was devastated as I thought about the possible outcome of macular degeneration. My thinking immediately brought me to the worst possible scenario. I envisioned the end of carving, skiing, and boating, and I saw myself having to hold onto my wife's elbow for the remainder of my life. I was not doing at all well with this thought. Education and beginning treatments helped me a great deal.

PART TWO

Risk Factors and Causes

What are the risk factors for age-related macular degeneration?

Are men or women more likely to get age-related macular degeneration?

I have a family history of macular degeneration. Is there anything I can do to avoid getting it myself?

More . . .

17. What are the risk factors for age-related macular degeneration?

The most important risk factor for age-related macular degeneration is age. Although macular degeneration can occur in patients younger than 50 years of age, it is uncommon. Numerous studies show that people over the age of 60 years are at greatest risk for development of macular degeneration. The risk continues to increase the older a person is, and studies have shown that it may be as high as 30% in those 75 years of age and older.

Current smokers have a two- to fourfold greater risk of developing the later stages of macular degeneration than nonsmokers.

Smoking is another consistent risk factor associated with the development of macular degeneration. Current smokers have a two- to fourfold greater risk of developing the later stages of macular degeneration than nonsmokers. Even after quitting, an increased risk persists for as long as 15 years—or even longer. However, the risk decreases with cessation of tobacco use. This decreased risk is even apparent in the first year of stopping. Smoking not only increases the risk of macular degeneration, but current or recent smokers cannot take the recommended vitamin supplement for macular degeneration prevention because beta-carotene, one of the vitamins in these supplements, increases the risk of lung cancer in smokers.

Family history is another strong risk factor. Patients with a first-degree relative who has macular degeneration have a two- to threefold greater risk of developing the disease than patients without first-degree relatives with macular degeneration.

In addition to family history, tremendous work with regard to macular degeneration and genetics has revealed that certain genes are strongly associated with macular degeneration. Patients who have particular variants of this gene have a much greater risk of developing the disease. One such variant involves the complement factor H gene, or CFH gene. The presence of this variant may account for almost 50% of all cases in the United States.

Other risk factors include race (Whites are more likely to lose vision from macular degeneration than African Americans), gender (women appear to be at greater risk than men), and obesity. Studies typically include these three factors as reasonably well-accepted causes associated with macular degeneration. Other characteristics, such as farsightedness, light iris color, sunlight exposure, and hypertension have been associated with macular degeneration in some studies, classifying these characteristics as possible risk factors. While any form of hypertension may be associated with increased risk of developing macular degeneration, uncontrolled hypertension (defined as blood pressure greater than 160/95 mm Hg) is associated with more of a risk.

18. What causes macular degeneration?

The exact causes of age-related macular degeneration are not known. Researchers and clinicians believe that the causes of macular degeneration are multifactorial, meaning there are a number of different factors that may contribute to the disease. Multiple studies have identified and continue to validate a hereditary or genetic predisposition to age-related macular degeneration; however, there also appears to be a contribution from environmental and nutritional factors. Risk factors associated with macular degeneration include older age, race (White), smoking, high intake of saturated fats, and exposure to sunlight. Some of these risks are discussed in the previous question, and others will be discussed in greater detail in subsequent questions.

Recent research with regard to genetic findings, such as the association of the CFH gene and macular degeneration, suggest a role of chronic inflammation in macular degeneration. CFH plays a role in controlling inflammation in the body, and its association with macular degeneration points to inflammation as contributing in some manner to macular degeneration. A number of researchers are focusing tremendous time and funding in an effort to learn about the role of inflammation, genetics, and macular degeneration.

19. Are men or women more likely to get age-related macular degeneration?

While many studies suggest women are more likely to get macular degeneration than men, gender remains an inconsistent risk factor. When the largest studies of age-related macular degeneration are reviewed and all of the results combined, it does appear as if there might be a slightly increased risk in women over men. This appears to be a true increase in risk and not simply related to the longer life expectancy of women relative to men.

20. Is smoking a risk factor for macular degeneration?

Smoking is clearly a risk factor for the development of age-related macular degeneration. It appears that smoking not only increases risk of developing macular degeneration, it also promotes its progression. In addition, smoking influences many other prevalent diseases that affect the elderly, including heart disease and stroke. Patients with macular degeneration who would like to actively alter their risk of progression should clearly take steps to stop smoking. Smoking represents one of the most modifiable risk factors associated with age-related macular degeneration. Stopping smoking does reduce the risk of developing macular degeneration; 20 years after stopping, the risk is similar to someone who never smoked. However, the benefits of stopping smoking may occur almost immediately, with a decreased risk of 6–7% within the first year.

21. Does age-related macular degeneration have a racial predilection?

Studies show that Whites are more likely to lose vision from age-related macular degeneration than are individuals of other races. Although macular degeneration is more common in Whites, it does occur in all races.

22. I have a family history of macular degeneration. Is there anything I can do to avoid getting it myself?

Although there is clearly a hereditary component to macular degeneration, having a family history does not guarantee that subsequent family members will acquire it. With regard to decreasing one's risk, at this time, there is no absolute means of preventing its onset. There are, however, actions that may prove beneficial. For instance, eating a well-balanced diet with foods rich in a source of **antioxidants**, such as spinach, collard greens, and kale, may be beneficial. Studies have shown that patients deficient in antioxidants have a higher risk of developing various stages of macular degeneration. Incorporating **omega-3 fatty acids** twice a week into one's diet may also be helpful. Although studies are ongoing as to whether or not these polyunsaturated fatty acids are beneficial in preventing macular degeneration, there appears to be a growing body of

Antioxidants

Substances that prevent oxidative damage in our body. For instance, spinach, collard greens, and kale are sources of antioxidants important in combating macular degeneration.

Eating a well-balanced diet with foods rich in a source of antioxidants, such as spinach, collard greens, and kale, may be beneficial.

Omega-3 fatty acids

A family of unsaturated fatty acids that may have health benefits, including reducing heart disease and depression. Oily fish such as salmon and tuna are excellent sources of omega-3 fatty acids.

proof that they are beneficial in other diseases such as cardiac disease and depression.

There is no proof that taking vitamin supplements is helpful for those without a certain degree of macular degeneration already present. In fact, the Age-Related Eye Disease Study (AREDS) did not show a benefit of supplemental antioxidants in patients with early stages of age-related macular degeneration. There is also no proof that protecting one's eyes from the sun will prevent the onset of macular degeneration; however, common sense dictates that this certainly would not hurt a patient and may, at some point, prove beneficial.

Nick's comment:

I was 60 years old when my macular degeneration was first diagnosed. At the age of 28, I became a certified ski instructor and was employed at Wildcat Mountain in Pinkham Notch, New Hampshire, opposite Mt. Washington. Being young and "cool," we thought we looked better without sunglasses (protection). I've been told that the glare of the sun bouncing off of the snow doubles the intensity of the reflection. I am sure this was not a benefit to my eyes.

23. Both of my parents have macular degeneration. Does this mean I will have it also?

Both parents having macular degeneration is not a guarantee that you will have it; however, there is clearly a hereditary component to macular degeneration. Recent research has found that variants of different genes are present in many, if not most, patients who have macular degeneration. The fact that one's parents have macular degeneration is suggestive that they may have one of the genes associated with macular degeneration, and therefore may have passed it on to their children. It is not, however, a certainty.

Nick's comment:

Knowing what I know now, I have tried to educate my three children, ages 27, 35, and 40 years old, as to how very critical eye exams are. Having glaucoma as well as macular degeneration raises my awareness for them. I reinforce the time factor always, meaning the sooner the better—time is of the essence. I encourage annual checkups, or more often if necessary.

24. Is it possible to modify the risk factors for age-related macular degeneration?

Certain risk factors may be affected by lifestyle changes. The most obvious one is discontinuing smoking, when applicable. Discontinuing smoking can show benefits almost immediately, with a decrease in the risk of developing wet macular degeneration occurring in the first year and decreasing further over the next 10–20 years. Other lifestyle changes that may be important include eating a healthy diet that includes **green leafy vegetables** high in antioxidants (such as spinach, collard greens, and kale) and also includes fish and almonds (both sources of omega-3 fatty acids, which have been associated with a decreased risk of macular degeneration). Since obesity may be a risk factor, and since there are associations between high blood pressure and possibly other vascular diseases, maintaining a normal blood pressure, exercising regularly, and attending to one's weight are reasonable recommendations.

Green leafy vegetables

Vegetables such as spinach, collard greens, and kale that are high in antioxidants. Lettuce is not high in such nutrients.

25. I also have cataracts. Are age-related macular degeneration and cataracts related?

The general consensus is that cataracts and macular degeneration are not related and that they develop independently of one another.

The general consensus is that cataracts and macular degeneration are not related and that they develop independently of one another. Numerous studies have looked at both, and the majority of these studies have not shown a relationship. Those studies that have shown any type of relationship have been contradictory, meaning one study has shown a relationship of one type of cataract and not another, and these findings have been completely reversed in other studies. When all of these data are pooled, it does not appear as if the two conditions are related; however, both are extremely common, and therefore patients commonly have both cataracts and age-related macular degeneration.

PART THREE

Dry Age-Related Macular Degeneration: What Is It, How Can I Recognize It, and What Can I Do About It?

How is dry macular degeneration diagnosed?

What are the early symptoms of dry macular degeneration?

I understand that new medicines are available to treat wet macular degeneration. Will these medicines also help my dry macular degeneration?

More . . .

Nick's comment:

Due to a published article written about my progress with treatment, people would call me with questions. I would explain the urgency of acting upon their problem. I would talk about the importance of seeing a retina specialist right away. Often they would recontact me 4–6 months later asking how I was doing. In turn I would ask the same and often the response was "a lot worse." Then, I would learn that they had not seen an ophthalmologist yet!

26. What is dry macular degeneration?

Dry macular degeneration is a disease of the macula in which the cells in the macula gradually break down, often leading to some degree of visual loss (see **Figure 4**). Dry macular degeneration is by far the more common type (versus wet macular degeneration), although of the two types, it is less likely to cause severe visual loss. Dry macular degeneration accounts for approximately 90% of all macular degeneration patients. The breakdown of the macular cells is believed to be due to impaired

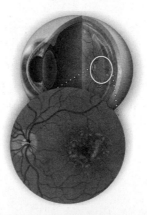

Figure 4   The retina with dry macular degeneration.

© 2009 www.JirehDesign.com. All rights reserved.

ability of certain cells in the macula to get rid of breakdown products. When we are younger, these products are easily taken care of, but as we get older, our ability to handle this process declines. Accumulation of these breakdown products leads to the formation of drusen, yellow deposits in the macula. Over time (years), it is hypothesized that drusen impair the normal transfer of nutrients between layers in the retina, resulting in macular damage and visual loss.

27. How is dry macular degeneration diagnosed?

Dry macular degeneration is diagnosed by your eye care provider based on a **dilated** examination of your retina. A number of characteristic findings can be seen. These include drusen, changes in the layer underneath the retina (pigmentary changes in the retinal pigment epithelium), and occasional blisterlike elevations of the retina. Drusen, which are described in the following question, are yellow deposits underneath the retina. They may be of varying size, shape, and consistency. The pigment changes in the layer underneath the retina consist of pigment clumping and pigment atrophy. These often give a salt-and-pepper–type appearance to the retina. The blisterlike elevations, called pigment epithelial detachments, can be noted on retinal examination, but often further diagnostic imaging is required to confirm their presence and to ensure that they are not associated with wet macular degeneration. Upon diagnosis, your eye care provider will often have photographs taken of your eye to document the current findings.

Occasionally, it may be important to differentiate dry from wet macular degeneration. This may require a dye test called a **fluorescein angiogram (FA)** (discussed in

Dilation

Enlargement of the pupils with eye drops.

Fluorescein angiogram (FA)

A diagnostic test in which dye is injected into a patient's arm, and then photographed as it travels to and through the blood vessels of the retina. It helps retina specialists to detect abnormalities, such as new blood vessels, in wet macular degeneration.

Optical coherence tomography (OCT)

A noninvasive diagnostic imaging technique of the eye in which detailed cross-sectional images of the retina are obtained.

Indocyanine green (ICG)

A dye test of the retina similar to fluorescein angiography but designed to evaluate the layer beneath the retina (the choroid). It is occasionally used to evaluate difficult or refractory cases of wet macular degeneration.

greater detail in Question 52). The angiogram is helpful in demonstrating leakage from wet macular degeneration. Another helpful test is **optical coherence tomography (OCT)** (discussed in Question 54). This test often shows fluid in the retina, another indication of wet macular degeneration (see **Figure 5**). In more difficult cases, a second dye test called **indocyanine green (ICG),** which shows somewhat different characteristics of the retina, may be ordered as well. It is often helpful for you and your family to review these findings with your ophthalmologist.

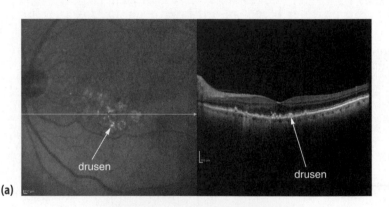

(a)

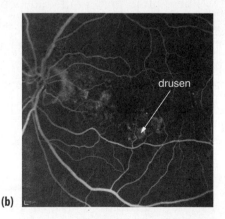

(b)

Figure 5   (a and b) Examples of dry macular degeneration OCT and FA.

28. My ophthalmologist told me I have a number of drusen in my retina. What are drusen, and how do they relate to macular degeneration?

Drusen are yellow deposits in the layer under the retina. They may be of various sizes, shapes, and consistencies. These characteristics help to determine a patient's risk for vision loss and/or progression to wet macular degeneration. Small, **hard drusen** are of least concern and, if the only findings, may not even represent age-related macular degeneration. Medium-sized drusen are typically associated with age-related macular degeneration. Drusen may be defined as "hard," in which they are well defined and have an almost crystalline appearance, or "**soft**," in which they are somewhat more amorphous and coalesce to form larger areas. Finally, large drusen are of greatest risk for vision loss or progression to wet macular degeneration.

Drusen represent breakdown products in the level underneath the retina. The **retinal pigment epithelium (RPE),** the layer underneath the retina, is responsible for the degradation of regular breakdown products in the normal functioning of the retina. Over time, the ability of the retinal pigment epithelium to perform these activities declines, and drusen and pigmentary changes are the end result.

29. What are the early symptoms of dry macular degeneration?

In the early stages of dry macular degeneration, patients are often **asymptomatic**. The earliest findings in dry macular degeneration, drusen and mild breakdown of the layer underneath the retina (the retinal

Hard drusen

Small, discrete, well-demarcated yellow deposits beneath the retina. Hard drusen are less likely to progress to more advanced stages of macular degeneration than soft drusen.

Soft drusen

Poorly demarcated, amorphous yellow deposits beneath the retina. Soft drusen are more likely to progress to advanced stages of macular degeneration than hard drusen.

Retinal pigment epithelium (RPE)

The layer of cells beneath or outside the retina that serves to nourish the retinal photoreceptors (the light-sensing cells of the retina) as well as to remove or digest toxic byproducts generated in the photoreceptors.

Asymptomatic

Without symptoms.

pigment epithelium), often go unnoticed. As these findings progress, patients may become aware of mild distortion or blurriness. Patients will often mistake these symptoms as being secondary to a **refractive error** (meaning they need a change in their glasses) or attribute them to cataracts. Patients often ignore early symptoms and only mention them to their eye care provider at their annual examination.

Refractive error

A focusing error of the eye that results in blurred vision. Hyperopia and myopia are examples of refractive errors.

30. What are the symptoms of more advanced dry macular degeneration?

While more advanced stages of dry macular degeneration can still be asymptomatic, this tends not to be the case. Patients often complain of blurring or distortion, which can affect their daily activities. Because many of these patients also have cataracts, the symptoms may be mistaken for those due solely to the cataract. Ocular examination with the patient's eye care provider often differentiates between the two conditions. As the dry macular degeneration continues to progress, mild distortion may turn into significant difficulty with reading or distance vision, and areas may even darken or blur out entirely. In addition, patients often require and become dependent on better or brighter lighting to perform their daily activities.

As the dry macular degeneration continues to progress, mild distortion may turn into significant difficulty with reading or distance vision, and areas may even darken or blur out entirely.

31. Why do my eyes have to be dilated at my regular follow-ups?

Macular degeneration is a disease of the retina. The retina is in the back of the eye, and the best method of examining the back of the eye is with a dilated retinal examination. Enlargement of the pupil offers the ophthalmologist the best view of the retina—one that is in stereovision, or three-dimensional. In addition, the dilated exam is ideal for any type of photography that the ophthalmologist feels is necessary to better evaluate the macula. In general, a dilated examination allows for the highest quality of imaging, which is often a necessary part of the examination. The dilation usually lasts several hours, typically 3 to 4, although in some patients it can last longer. It is often recommended that patients bring sunglasses to the examination to be more comfortable when the examination is completed. To avoid having to drive with dilated eyes upon completion of the exam, many patients bring family members or friends to the examination.

Nick's comment:

The result of dilation for me was blurry vision and was no fun. But, I found that taking a nap or just shutting my eyes for an hour or so was a great help. I recommend not driving!

32. Will changing my glasses help improve my vision?

The damage that occurs from macular degeneration is to the retina. Damage to the retina is not correctable by changes in glasses. Glasses correct for various refractive errors such as being **nearsighted**, **farsighted**, or having an **astigmatism** (an abnormal curvature to the eye). While a change in glasses will not improve the vision that is damaged from macular degeneration, maximizing one's glasses can help to improve the overall vision. Such adjustments do not correct for the macular degeneration, but they do ensure that any refractive error is appropriately corrected. If you or your ophthalmologist is not certain, it is reasonable to undergo a refraction to see if it helps with the quality of vision.

Nearsighted

An abnormality of the eye in which the eye cannot focus properly on distant objects.

Farsighted

An abnormality of the eye in which it cannot focus properly on near objects.

Astigmatism

A condition in which abnormal shape of either a person's cornea or lens (or both) result in blurred vision.

33. I understand that new medicines are available to treat wet macular degeneration. Will these medicines also help my dry macular degeneration?

Anti-VEGF agents, such as Lucentis (ranibizumab) or Avastin (bevacizumab), address the new blood vessel growth associated with wet macular degeneration. They also help eliminate the fluid leakage that occurs in association with the new vessel growth. Both of these effects are important in the treatment of wet macular degeneration. Unfortunately, they do not impact dry macular degeneration. The degeneration, or breakdown, of the retina associated with dry macular degeneration, appears to be driven by other factors. These factors are being heavily studied in labs and clinical trials.

34. How fast does dry macular degeneration progress?

Dry macular degeneration tends to be a slowly progressive disease, with subtle changes occurring over time. These changes may be noticed by the patient with gradually decreasing vision. Patients may also recognize these changes due to other symptoms, including gradually increasing distortion or gradual impairment of the ability to read.

In less common cases, sudden changes may occur. These sudden changes may be the culmination of a more gradual process, resulting in the involvement of a critical part of the macula. For instance, if dry macular degeneration began near, but not in, the center of the macula has occurred around the center of the macula and finally spreads to involve the center, the involvement of this critical area may cause immediate changes in vision. Therefore, even though the overall process has progressed slowly, the involvement of this area will result in a sudden change, and this change may be dramatic. This is most often the case when geographic atrophy, an advanced form of dry macular degeneration, occurs and involves the center.

It is impossible, however, for an ophthalmologist to predict with any degree of certainty the speed of progression or the rate of visual loss. One eye may progress rapidly with loss of central vision while the other eye remains relatively stable with preservation of central vision. As described in Question 38, numerous researchers are studying investigational approaches to dry macular degeneration in order to prevent progression (either to more severe stages of dry disease or to wet disease). Many of these approaches are promising, and researchers are hopeful that breakthroughs will occur in the near future.

35. How can I monitor my macular degeneration?

The best way to monitor changes in macular degeneration is to establish a regular schedule of checking your central vision. A regular schedule can vary depending upon one's comfort level. A typical schedule is to check your vision anywhere from one to several times a week. This can be done using a block of squares called an **Amsler grid**, which is discussed in the next question, or using any object that has a regular pattern on it. For instance, a window with regular panes, a floor with regular tiles, or a picture with a series of straight lines will work best. A pattern of straight lines is most beneficial, as one of the early symptoms of wet macular degeneration is distortion of straight lines. It is best to establish a baseline of the object that is used to monitor your vision and to report any changes as

Amsler grid

A grid of vertical and horizontal straight lines in a square with a dot in the center designed as a screening test for detecting early macular abnormalities, such as wet macular degeneration.

soon as they occur. Each eye should be checked separately by covering the fellow eye during checking.

Many patients monitor their vision by a regular daily activity. For instance, if they routinely read the newspaper, which has relatively small print, they will note changes in their ability to do so. If increasing difficulty is apparent, they will schedule an appointment with their eye care provider. One company is currently investigating a home device that may help patients to monitor their macular degeneration by testing on a more sensitive computer program that measures vision differently, and presumably more accurately, than an Amsler grid. The device, called the Preferential Hyperacuity Perimeter may be available for home use in the not-too-distant future.

36. What is an Amsler grid?

An Amsler grid (**Figure 6**) is helpful at detecting changes in one's central vision. The grid consists of a square with a pattern of smaller squares contained within it. It is designed to be held a comfortable reading distance from the person using it. Changes to vision are often detected as areas where the lines are no longer straight, but are bent or distorted, or where the lines are actually absent. When used regularly, an Amsler grid may help patients detect early changes in their macular degeneration. In general, the earlier changes are detected, the more likely it is that treatment will be effective, especially if the changes are due to wet macular degeneration.

When using the grid, each eye should be checked separately by covering the fellow eye. Patients are instructed to look at the central dot. If they see the central dot, they should continue looking at it while trying to see all four corners and all four sides of the chart.

In general, the earlier changes are detected, the more likely it is that treatment will be effective, especially if the changes are due to wet macular degeneration.

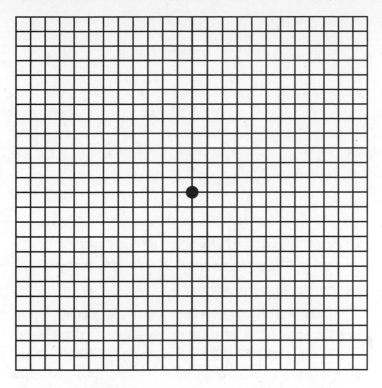

Figure 6   Amsler grid.

Do they appear straight? Are the lines inside the chart all present, and are they all straight? If not, one's eye care provider should be contacted immediately. If upon examination it is determined that wet macular degeneration has not occurred, then the changes noted on the Amsler grid should be considered one's baseline, and only additional changes should be reported.

Amsler grid testing is not foolproof, and subtle or significant disease progression may go undetected. Therefore, regular examinations, as determined by your eye care provider, are important. These exams may vary from every 3 months to annually, based upon the stage of your dry macular degeneration and the risk of progression.

Nick's comment:

It was pointed out to me in the beginning that time was of the essence. Today I am so pleased that I listened to and acted on that advice. My doctor had given me the Amsler grid, which is very easy to use, and I used it as a bookmark in whatever book I was reading. That way, I was able to look at the grid daily and detect any changes in my vision immediately

37. My doctor told me I have dry macular degeneration, but my eyes are always tearing. Does this mean I actually have wet macular degeneration?

The "dry" refers to the type of macular degeneration, not the state of lubrication of the superficial front part of the eye. Dry macular degeneration defines the characteristics of the macular degeneration. Macular degeneration is a disease of the retina, which is in the back of the eye. Tearing is a result of an abnormality of either tear production or tear drainage, both of which relate to the front of the eye. Increased tear production can be the result of irritation in the front of the eye, abnormalities of the corneal surface (the cornea is the front clear part of the eye), or even dry eyes. Dry eyes often result in irritation and trigger reflex tearing, which can actually result in increased tearing despite the overall presence of dry eye syndrome.

Normal tearing is controlled by the eye and increases or decreases based upon a feedback mechanism in the eye that responds to the amount of tears that are present. If irritation is not relieved by normal tearing, reflex tearing kicks in and adds additional tears to the surface of the eye to help lubricate it. Unfortunately, reflex tearing is not regulated by a feedback mechanism like normal tearing, and once stimulated, proceeds unchecked, often resulting in over-tearing.

Abnormalities of tear drainage may result from obstructions of the duct that removes tears from the eye, or from abnormalities of lid position. Appropriate lid apposition to the eye is necessary to have normal tear drainage.

All of these problems are related to the front of the eye and have no relation whatsoever to whether a person has dry or wet macular degeneration. If these symptoms are bothersome, contact your ophthalmologist for further evaluation.

38. Are there treatments for dry macular degeneration?

At this time, the recommendations for patients with dry macular degeneration revolve around nutrition and vitamin supplementation. Supplements may help to prevent progression of dry macular degeneration, as discussed in other questions in this book. There are no treatments per se to reverse either the anatomic changes or visual changes of dry macular degeneration. Fortunately, there is a great deal of research currently focused on dry macular degeneration. Past studies, which were not successful, included applying a pattern of laser to patients who had intermediate dry macular degeneration, blood transfusions to try to remove toxic elements that were thought to possibly lead to dry macular degeneration from the blood, and a **periocular** injection of a steroidlike derivative to prevent progression from dry to wet macular degeneration. None of these treatments proved beneficial.

Periocular

Around, but not in, the eye. Periocular injections are outside the eye, unlike intravitreal injections, which are in the eye.

However, numerous innovative approaches to dry macular degeneration are being tested in humans, including treatments to prevent the dry disease from progressing to wet macular degeneration, as well as treatments to prevent progression of the dry disease to more advanced stages of the dry disease (geographic atrophy). Vitamin supplementation, which is discussed more extensively in Part 4, may help to prevent progression from intermediate stages of dry macular degeneration to more advanced disease (geographic atrophy or wet macular degeneration). Other approaches currently under investigation include preventing buildup of toxic breakdown products that lead to drusen development, treatment to induce drusen regression or disappearance with the hope that this prevents development of advanced macular degeneration, and control of inflammation to limit drusen development or progression. Treatments are even being investigated that will limit or prevent further progression of atrophy for patients who have already developed various stages of geographic atrophy. Hopefully, breakthroughs will occur over the next several years, allowing clinicians to slow, stop, or prevent dry macular degeneration altogether.

PART FOUR

Vitamin Supplements and Diet

Are vitamin supplements recommended for all patients with age-related macular degeneration? Even if they aren't recommended for my stage of macular degeneration, will it hurt me to take them?

Do vitamins reverse dry macular degeneration?

Does eating fish help reduce macular degeneration?

More . . .

39. I often hear of the AREDS study or formulation. What is the AREDS formulation?

AREDS, or the Age-Related Eye Disease Study, was a large study involving more than 4700 patients that investigated the benefits of vitamin supplementation with respect to preventing the progression of dry macular degeneration. This study was sponsored by the National Eye Institute (a branch of the National Institutes of Health). The study showed that patients at high risk of developing advanced stages of macular degeneration lowered their risk by about 25% when using a specific combination of antioxidants and zinc. Patients were considered at high risk of progression if they had intermediate dry macular degeneration (defined by the presence of certain numbers of drusen of a particular size), wet macular degeneration, or geographic atrophy in one eye but not the other. The combination of nutrients also decreased the risk of vision loss by 19%.

The daily amounts in the AREDS formulation are 500 mg of vitamin C, 400 IU of vitamin E, 15 mg of beta-carotene, and 80 mg of zinc (as zinc oxide). The formulation also includes 2 mg of copper (as cupric oxide) to prevent copper deficiency anemia, a condition that may occur with high levels of zinc supplementation (see **Table 1**). It should be emphasized that daily use of the AREDS supplements is not a cure for macular degeneration; rather it is a treatment that helps to prevent progression and visual loss.

Daily use of the AREDS supplements is not a cure for macular degeneration; rather it is a treatment that helps to prevent progression and visual loss.

Table 1   The Breakdown of AREDS Vitamin Supplements

Vitamin C	Vitamin E	Beta Carotene	Zinc	Copper
500 mg	400 IU	15 mg	80 mg	2 mg

40. Is there a difference between vitamin supplements?

There are numerous eye vitamins available. Those recommended for patients with age-related macular degeneration are supplements that have the AREDS formulation (see Question 39). To be fair, it is not known whether other formulations may be comparable or even better, but the best and most complete research available is that of the AREDS formulation; therefore, it is the AREDS formulation that is recommended by the American Academy of Ophthalmology. Several manufacturers make an AREDS formulation, and this is usually stated on the outside of the bottle; however, if you have any questions, your pharmacist will be able to direct you to an AREDS formulation.

41. Are vitamin supplements recommended for all patients with age-related macular degeneration? Even if they aren't recommended for my stage of macular degeneration, will it hurt me to take them?

Vitamin supplementation is recommended for patients with a specific stage of macular degeneration. The patients who have been shown to benefit from vitamin supplementation are those with intermediate dry macular degeneration and those with wet or advanced macular degeneration in one eye and not their fellow eye. The intermediate stage is defined by many drusen of medium size, or one or more large drusen. Those without any evidence of macular degeneration, or with only early dry macular degeneration, have not been shown to benefit from supplementation. Some patients with early dry macular degeneration progressed to the intermediate stage during the AREDS study. The AREDS supplementation did not appear to slow this progression.

Patients with macular degeneration should consult their eye care provider, who will help them determine whether or not they should take the vitamins.

One should definitely be careful about taking high-dose nutritional supplements without consulting a physician. While many nutritional supplements are harmless, numerous studies have shown that some may cause serious side effects. For instance, zinc in the concentrations recommended for the over-the-counter supplement may lead to copper deficiency anemia. This concern is addressed by the addition of copper to the AREDS formulation. Studies have also shown that beta-carotene use in smokers increases their risk of developing lung cancer. As a result, there are smokers' formulations that don't use the beta-carotene. Vitamin E use has been associated with increased death rates when used in high doses. This risk was not seen in the AREDS trial.

It is recommended that patients consult their primary care physician prior to taking high-dose vitamin supplements. It is wrong to assume that because a nutrient may have beneficial effects with regard to one disease, the nutrient is harmless. Its use may have negative effects with regard to other disease states, such as those described here, or it may impede the body's absorption of other important nutrients. These types of effects are typically not apparent until large, carefully conducted trials in thousands of patients, such as the AREDS trial, are performed.

42. Do vitamins reverse dry macular degeneration?

Vitamins do not reverse dry macular degeneration. Vitamins are not a cure for macular degeneration. Studies have shown, however, that vitamins may be helpful in preventing progression of dry macular degeneration and/or limiting vision loss. When a specific combination of antioxidants and zinc is taken daily, a modest benefit with regard to progression of disease and prevention of vision loss has been documented; therefore, vitamin supplementation is recommended for certain patients with dry macular degeneration.

43. Are the AREDS vitamins helpful to those who do not have evidence of macular degeneration?

At this time, there is no evidence that the AREDS supplements are protective or beneficial for those without evidence of macular degeneration. Family members of patients with macular degeneration often ask if taking the AREDS supplements will help protect them from developing macular degeneration. This benefit has not been demonstrated. Patients who entered the AREDS trial with early dry macular degeneration experienced progression to intermediate dry disease without evidence of slowing. Therefore, the AREDS supplements are not recommended for anyone who does not have at least intermediate age-related macular degeneration or evidence of wet macular degeneration in one eye. A reasonable precautionary step is to eat a well-balanced diet with green leafy vegetables that are high in antioxidants. In addition, lower amounts of antioxidants are typical components of daily multivitamins.

44. Do I need a prescription for AREDS supplements?

AREDS supplements, like other types of vitamins, including daily multivitamins, are over-the-counter and do not require a prescription; however, it is strongly recommended that patients notify or discuss with their primary care provider their intent to take the AREDS multivitamins. AREDS formulations do have higher than normally recommended amounts of antioxidants, and your primary care provider will want to be aware of this.

45. Many of the over-the-counter eye supplements advertise the inclusion of lutein. Does lutein help to prevent macular degeneration or its progression, and should I take it?

Lutein

An antioxidant found in green leafy vegetables that may be helpful in preventing or slowing macular degeneration.

Zeaxanthin

A type of pigment located in the retina that has antioxidant properties.

Lutein is a pigment in the macula that along with another pigment (**zeaxanthin**), is believed to protect the macula from damaging effects of blue light. Lutein has been the focus of studies over the past several years, the majority of which suggest a benefit with regard to decreasing the risk of macular degeneration. The recommended dosage is 6–20 mg/day. Lutein can also be obtained in one's diet. It is present in green leafy vegetables like spinach, kale, collard greens, and broccoli. It is also present in relatively high amounts in corn. Studies demonstrating a causal relationship have not yet been reported.

AREDS II is a current clinical trial evaluating an antioxidant regimen with and without lutein, zeaxanthin, and omega-3 fatty acids.

46. Does eating green leafy vegetables help reduce macular degeneration?

Green leafy vegetables are sources of lutein and zeaxanthin carotenoids that are concentrated in the eye and may play a protective role against age-related macular degeneration. Studies have not confirmed conclusively that eating green leafy vegetables helps to prevent macular degeneration; however, patients who have

Table 2   Sources High in Lutein and Xeaxanthan

Foods High in Lutein and Zeaxanthin Based on Levels per 100-gram Serving	
Kale: raw- Lutein + Zeaxanthin	39551mcg
Turnip Greens: raw- Lutein + Zeaxanthin	12824mcg
Spinach: raw- Lutein + Zeaxanthin	12197mcg
Collard Greens: raw- Lutein + Zeaxanthin	8932mcg
Broccoli: raw- Lutein + Zeaxanthin	1403mcg
Corn: sweet, yellow, raw- Lutein + Zeaxanthin	644mcg
Squash: summer, crookneck and straightneck, raw- Lutein + Zeaxanthin	290mcg
Carrots: raw- Lutein + Zeaxanthin	256mcg
Tomatoes: red, ripe, raw, year-round average- Lutein + Zeaxanthin	123mcg

Source: www.nutritiondata.com

reported eating low levels of green leafy vegetables do seem to be at greater risk. Lutein and zeaxanthin may help to absorb blue light from the sun's rays and may act as antioxidants. Green leafy vegetables include spinach, collard greens, and kale. Of note, corn also is reasonably high in lutein (see **Table 2**).

47. Does eating fish help reduce macular degeneration?

Several studies have suggested that eating fish and other foods high in omega-3 fatty acids is associated with a reduced risk of developing both early and late age-related macular degeneration. Omega-3 fatty acids are antioxidants that protect cells from sun, aging, or environmental damage. Studies have suggested that eating oily fish at least once a week may be associated with a decreased risk of macular degeneration. Eating two servings of fish per week may provide an even higher protective benefit. Additional benefits to eating such fish include potential decreased risk of cancers and perhaps even some forms of heart disease.

As the answer to this question is not clearly known, the AREDS II trial is evaluating the benefit of omega-3 fatty acids with respect to macular degeneration. Omega-3 fatty acids are found in oily cold water fish like salmon, trout, and tuna. Flax seeds and walnuts are also rich in omega-3 fatty acids.

48. Do bilberries, blueberries, or various nutritional supplements help with macular degeneration?

Bilberry

A dark, edible berry (similar to a blueberry) that has antioxidant activity.

Small studies have suggested **bilberry** may be helpful in preventing macular degeneration occurrence or progression. It has not, however, been the focus of a randomized, controlled trial (the type of trial that is most helpful and objective in determining a new treatment's efficacy). A theory exists regarding bilberry's positive effect on night vision, as allegedly proven when it was used by Britain's Royal Air Force pilots during World War II. This finding has not been corroborated in subsequent studies.

Blueberries are also believed to have antioxidant properties and may also be of benefit in preventing or slowing macular degeneration. However, blueberries, like bilberries, have not been evaluated in randomized clinical trials. This lack of study does not mean that either blueberries or bilberries are not beneficial, but simply that they have not been subjected to the same scrutiny as AREDS supplements; therefore we cannot make definitive recommendations. Without such evidence, it seems reasonable to suggest that one's diet be rich in such foods, but the administration of supplements without more data carries potential risks.

PART FIVE

Wet Age–Related Macular Degeneration: What Is It, How Will I Know if I Have It, Can It Be Treated?

What is wet macular degeneration?

What is a fluorescein angiogram?

Why do the lines appear wavy or crooked from wet macular degeneration?

More . . .

49. What is wet macular degeneration?

Wet macular degeneration (**Figure 7**) is an advanced form of macular degeneration in which new, abnormal blood vessels grow beneath or into the retina or the layers directly below the retina. In some instances, these new blood vessels actually originate from within the retina, a process referred to as retinal angiomatous proliferation, or RAP. The growth of these abnormal blood vessels is the eye's attempt to repair the effects of aging, sun exposure, inflammation, or other sources of damage to the eye. Unfortunately, these new vessels

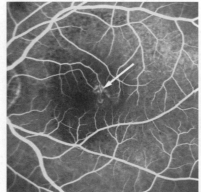
(a)

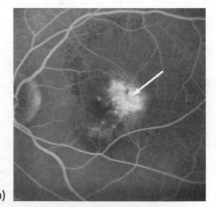
(b)

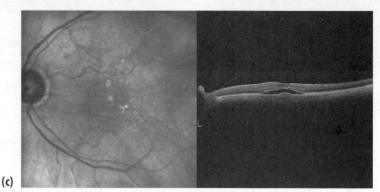
(c)

Figure 7 Examples of wet advanced macular degeneration OCT and FA. (a) Early phase of a fluorescein angiogram showing early leakage (arrow) secondary to new vessels of wet macular degeneration. (b) Late phase of the FA showing increased leakage (arrow). (c) OCT showing accumulation of fluid beneath the retina, a common finding in patients with macular degeneration. (See Question 27 also.)

are anything but helpful. These abnormal blood vessels are fragile and often leak fluid and blood beneath and into the retina. The fluid and blood lead to an abnormal contour of the retina and cause the distortion that one often notes as the initial symptom of wet macular degeneration. The greater the leakage, the greater the distortion and/or visual loss.

Early in the process, treatment with intraocular injections of anti-VEGF agents (discussed more extensively in Part 6) may result in stabilization and even significant visual recovery. With time, the effects of the leakage can lead to scarring and atrophy (loss of normal tissues), with irreversible vision loss. Prior to the discovery and use of anti-VEGF injections, clinicians differentiated the various types of wet macular degeneration based upon fluorescein angiographic characteristics (see Question 52). This differentiation was important, as only certain types of wet macular degeneration responded to the various therapies. The growths of new blood vessels were characterized as classic, occult, or a combination of the two. The classic type of pattern was more likely to respond to therapy and, in fact, was the only one to be approved for certain approaches. Fortunately, the newer treatments are more versatile with respect to treating the different patterns of leakage, and the different patterns are expected to respond to treatment.

Nick's comment:

My experience was definitely observing horizontal lines as wavy. I probably lived with this, knowing what I know now, for too long, thinking that it would probably go away on its own. I also found that during this period, much stronger lighting was very important to me. Little did I know that I should have sought professional advice immediately.

50. What are the symptoms of wet macular degeneration?

The most common symptom of wet macular degeneration is distorted vision.

The most common symptom of wet macular degeneration is distorted vision. This can be most easily appreciated when staring at objects that have a series of straight lines such as a windowpane, tiles, or the edge of a door. Another means of detecting this distortion is with an Amsler grid. The area of the retina affected by wet macular degeneration will no longer have the proper orientation or smoothness to allow the brain to interpret the line as being straight. It will therefore be seen as a curved or bumpy line. This visual distortion may be very subtle at first and hard to detect. In fact, the brain is quite capable of ignoring such subtle symptoms. However, as the wet macular degeneration worsens (i.e., as more leakage or bleeding occurs), the distortion becomes readily apparent (see **Figure 8**).

Additional symptoms include blurred or absent central vision. Bleeding can actually result in a dark or blind spot in the visual field and, depending upon the area of involvement, may entirely block a patient's central vision. Patients may realize these problems when staring at friends' or family members' faces and noting that parts of their faces can only be recognized by tilting or changing their eye position. This symptom may also be detected due to difficulty reading the headlines or smaller print of a newspaper, or due to difficulty following the headlines or small tickertape print at the bottom of a TV. If patients recognize these symptoms, they should contact their eye care provider immediately.

Nick's comment:

After being diagnosed with wet AMD, I continued to repeatedly watch the horizontal lines on my neighbor's house for a wavy effect. I continued this for some time after

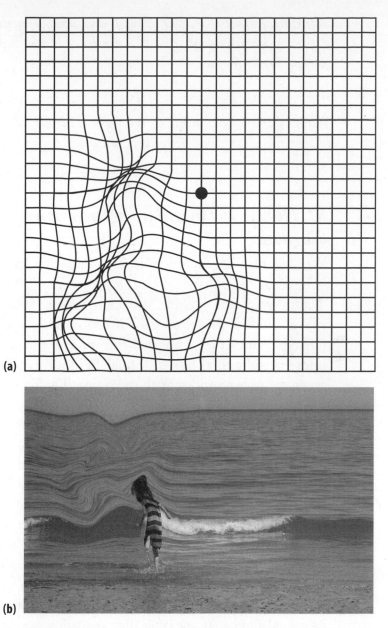

(a)

(b)

Figure 8 With advanced wet macular degeneration, (a) the Amsler grid and (b) everyday scenery will look distorted.

receiving Lucentis. In this way, I was able to mentally track my improvement. Also the Amsler grid was amazingly effective for me.

I live on the ocean and chose a permanent large nautical harbor buoy with a blinking red light. This helped me to determine clearly my levels of vision. I still watch it today.

51. How is wet macular degeneration diagnosed?

Wet macular degeneration is first suspected by your ophthalmologist based on symptoms you may describe. These symptoms include distorted vision, decreased vision, blurred vision, or loss of central vision. Upon dilated examination, your eye care provider may note intra- or subretinal blood, retinal fluid, or a grayish-green membrane underneath the retina. These findings are all highly suggestive of wet macular degeneration. Upon noting these abnormalities, your eye care provider, if not a retina specialist, will refer you to a retina specialist. Your retina specialist will then likely order a fluorescein angiogram. A fluorescein angiogram, described in Question 52, is a dye test that helps diagnose vascular diseases in the retina, such as wet macular degeneration. The retina specialist will also likely order a test known as optical coherence tomography, or OCT. The OCT, described in Question 54, gives a cross-sectional image of the retina, and it helps to show areas of retinal fluid that are typically noted in wet macular degeneration.

Nick's comment:

I developed glaucoma a few years prior to AMD and went routinely for pressure checks. I understand that AMD and glaucoma are two separate diseases. I just happen to have both. During my routine eye exam, something alerted my doctor to refer me to a retina specialist. That is when I met Dr. Heier.

52. What is a fluorescein angiogram?

A fluorescein angiogram is a dye test that helps to diagnose and characterize diseases of the retina (see **Figure 9**). Fluorescein is a dye that is injected into a vein in your arm and then travels throughout the blood vessels in

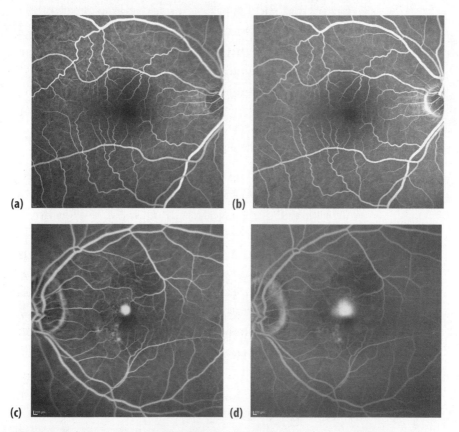

(a)　　　　　　　　　　　(b)

(c)　　　　　　　　　　　(d)

Figure 9　Examples of fluorescein angiograms. (a) Early phase of angiogram in normal retina. (b) Late phase of FA in normal retina. Note no leakage (increase in white dye as compared to (c) and (d)). (c) Early phase of FA showing leakage secondary to wet macular degeneration. (d) Later phase of FA showing increased leakage.

Wet Age-Related Macular Degeneration

your body, illuminating the blood vessels when exposed to a certain type of light. As the dye reaches the vessels in the eye, a camera photographs the eye. The fluorescein dye is seen in the normal vessels in the eye, but it is also seen in abnormal vessels or other types of disease states.

Macular degeneration is characterized by certain fluorescein angiographic findings, such as leakage from the abnormal blood vessels, and the size and site of the leakage can be detailed with this testing. Fluorescein angiography is commonly performed in newly diagnosed macular degeneration; it is often repeated when changes occur such as sudden vision loss or sudden onset of distorted vision. Retina specialists may also use fluorescein angiography to help make treatment decisions, such as when to hold or restart intraocular injections.

53. Are there any risks or side effects of fluorescein angiography?

There are side effects and risks to fluorescein angiography. After fluorescein dye is injected into your arm, your skin will turn a yellowish color for several hours. In addition, fluorescein is removed from the body by the kidneys and excreted in the urine. It turns the urine dark orange or yellow for about 24 hours.

Approximately 5% of patients who undergo fluorescein angiography experience the acute onset of nausea. This side effect occurs roughly 30–60 seconds into the test and usually passes quickly. An even smaller percentage of patients will actually experience vomiting. Again, this typically passes quickly.

Allergic reactions to fluorescein dye are uncommon but do occur. Symptoms may include itching, a skin rash, or a funny sensation in the throat. More serious allergic reactions are rare but have been reported, including breathing difficulties, chest tightness, and, in extremely rare cases, death. The risk of a severe allergic reaction associated with fluorescein dye is roughly 1 in 250,000.

Nick's comment:

I have had many fluorescein angiograms with no side effects.

54. What is optical coherence tomography (OCT)?

Optical coherence tomography (**Figure 10**) is an imaging technique that allows cross-sectional scans of the retina.

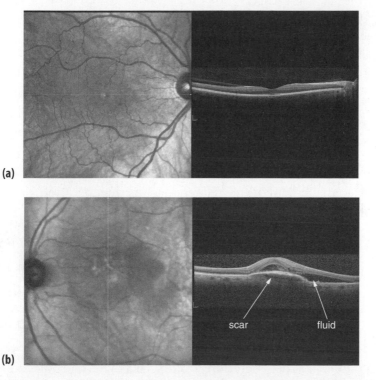

Figure 10   Examples of OCTs. (a) Normal retina. (b) A retina with wet advanced macular degeneration.

This technique utilizes light that is directed onto the tissue and reflects to form a pattern, similar to the process of ultrasound. The images obtained from OCT actually look like specimens of tissue that have been surgically cut and photographed. This technique has allowed **retina specialists** to manage age-related macular degeneration in a noninvasive manner with greater ability to interpret treatment responses. Recent advances in OCT have further added to clinicians' abilities to follow treatment. OCT has become so important to retina specialists that it is by far the most common diagnostic test ordered in the ongoing management of wet macular degeneration. While fluorescein angiography is critical for the initial diagnosis and at other points throughout treatment, OCT is the most common test utilized.

While fluorescein angiography is critical for the initial diagnosis and at other points throughout treatment, OCT is the most common test utilized.

55. Is there a limit to the number of OCTs a patient can undergo?

There is no limit to the number of OCTs a patient can have. The diagnostic tool utilized in OCT light poses no risk, either to the patient's eye or systemically. The beauty of this test lies in its noninvasive nature; therefore patients can have unlimited OCTs without any risk. This technique has become a critical component of the management of age-related macular degeneration.

56. Why do the lines appear wavy or crooked from wet macular degeneration?

When the macula is in its normal configuration (i.e., when it has its normal curve in the back of the eye), images that are seen by the macula are transmitted to the brain and recognized as being straight. When wet macular degeneration occurs, leakage and bleeding underneath the macula distort the normal architecture of the macula. Instead of having its normal curves, there will be areas that are elevated and irregular. An image that is now projected onto the macula is interpreted by the brain as being bumpy or irregular because the brain is not capable of differentiating an irregular or bumpy image from an irregular or bumpy macula. Therefore, the brain perceives any abnormality in the macula contour as an irregular or bumpy image.

Another common complaint is that images in the affected eye seem smaller than in the unaffected eye. This distortion is due to the photoreceptor cells, the cells in the macula that sense light and send an impulse to the brain, being distorted or swollen in such a way that fewer of them occupy a given space. For instance, if it normally took five cells to cover a certain area and, because of blood and fluid in and around the cells, only three are now able to occupy the same space, then the brain will interpret an image covering that same space as only being three cells big instead of five. The image is the same size, but the brain will think it is smaller because it only is touching three cells rather than five. Often, this distortion improves with successful treatment of wet macular degeneration; however, it rarely improves back to normal. Usually there is some mild persistent abnormality.

57. Why are some letters missing when I try to read?

Macular degeneration does not typically affect the retina in a symmetric or even pattern. Small areas, or even large areas, may be severely affected, while adjacent areas are minimally affected or not affected at all (see **Figure 11**). Therefore, when looking at a book or reading a sign, damaged areas may appear distorted or totally absent, while adjacent areas or less affected or unaffected areas may appear normal. If one side of the retina is more affected

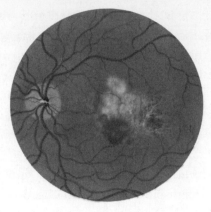

Figure 11   A retina with wet advanced macular degeneration.
© 2009 www.JirehDesign.com. All rights reserved.

than another it may be obvious when reading a book; the left side of the page may be easily seen, but as the eyes track to the right side of the page it may become more difficult to follow the sentence. Patients may adapt to these abnormalities and learn to move their head or eyes in a manner that maximizes their ability to read without disruption. Other patients may benefit from a low vision evaluation or vision rehabilitation evaluation in which they may be taught to adapt to the change by utilizing certain techniques or devices.

58. What does fluid in the retina mean? Is that the same as bleeding?

Fluid in the retina refers to leakage from the abnormal blood vessels associated with wet macular degeneration. While this is different from bleeding, the abnormal blood vessels can leak either fluid or blood, and sometimes leak both. Both are indicative of wet macular degeneration. While both are damaging, fluid may be

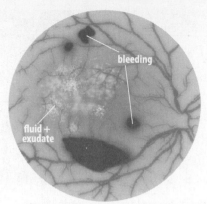

Figure 12   A retina with wet advanced macular degeneration showing leakage and bleeding.

less damaging, as fluid often reabsorbs easier and/or faster and the visual deficit from fluid is not as dense as that from blood (see **Figure 12**).

The presence or absence of fluid is the characteristic finding followed by OCT. Resolution of fluid, as monitored by OCT, is related to a patient's response to therapy and/or spontaneous improvement (see **Figure 13**). Recurrence of fluid or discovery of new fluid is often an indication for treatment, either initiation of treatment for the first time or retreatment after a period of observation. Fluorescein angiography provides critical information about leakage and is often helpful in the initial diagnosis of wet macular degeneration, but it does not provide quantitative measurements of the fluid that is present at a given time like OCT does. Fluorescein angiography is ordered far less frequently than OCT; typically when difficult treatment decisions are being considered, such as whether it is safe to hold treatment or why the treatment response is suboptimal.

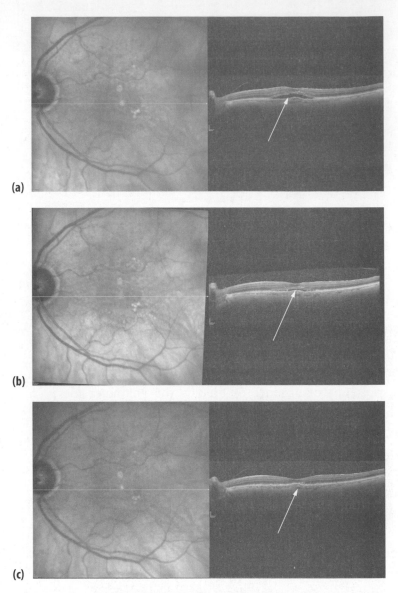

(a)

(b)

(c)

Figure 13 This series of OCTs shows an OCT of a wet AMD patient prior to treatment and responding to treatment. (a) An OCT showing significant fluid under the retina that is the result of new, untreated, wet macular degeneration (arrow) (b) Decreased fluid following a single injection of anti-VEGF therapy (arrow). (c) Complete resolution of fluid under the retina (arrow) following several anti-VEGF injections.

59. What is vascular endothelial growth factor (VEGF)?

Vascular endothelial growth factor, or VEGF, is a substance made by cells in the body that stimulates new blood vessel growth (see **Figure 14**). It also increases leakiness, or permeability, of blood vessels. Prior to being born, when we are developing in the womb, VEGF is important to blood vessel growth. VEGF is still believed to have important roles after we are born; however, in the eye, at least one type of VEGF causes abnormal blood vessel growth. VEGF is believed to be triggered or stimulated by various factors, such as poor oxygenation, inflammation, and cancer. The scientific recognition of VEGF as a major factor in the growth of new blood vessels associated with macular degeneration has led to the major breakthroughs in treatment with anti-VEGF therapy (**Figure 15**), such as Lucentis and Avastin (see Part 6).

Vascular endothelial growth factor (VEGF)

A growth factor produced by various tissues in the body in response to various stimuli. In the eye, VEGF is a major factor involved in wet macular degeneration and stimulates the growth of new blood vessels seen in this disease.

Wet Age-Related Macular Degeneration

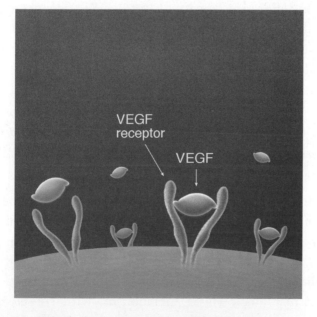

Figure 14   VEGF binding to a receptor on a cell in the retina.

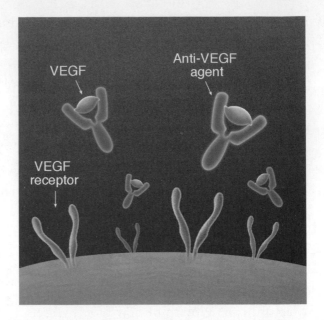

Figure 15   Anti-VEGF agents blocking VEGF from binding to receptor.

VEGF works by binding to receptors on certain cells of the body and then triggering the receptors to initiate an action. In the case of wet macular degeneration, the triggered action is the growth of new blood vessels, as well as increased permeability (leakiness) of vessels and the signaling of other cells to come to the area.

60. I have diabetes. Is macular degeneration related to my diabetes? Will it affect my diabetes?

Age-related macular degeneration and **diabetic retinopathy** (see **Figure 16**) are two distinct entities. They are not related, nor are they believed to impact one another. Diabetic retinopathy is secondary to **diabetes mellitus,** a vascular disease characterized by abnormal blood sugar metabolism, with subsequent negative effects on several body systems. The most

Diabetic retinopathy

Eye disease in which damage occurs secondary to high levels of blood sugar. Signs of diabetic retinopathy include retinal hemorrhages, cotton-wool spots, exudates, swelling, and new blood vessel growth.

Diabetes mellitus

A disease in which abnormally high blood sugars lead to damage of various organs of the body, including the heart, kidneys, and eyes.

common side effects of diabetes mellitus include kidney problems, neurologic problems, and, unfortunately, eye problems. Early eye problems manifest as small hemorrhages in the retina, mini-infarcts in the retina called **cotton-wool spots**, and transient visual blurring due to shrinking and swelling of one's lens. More advanced retinopathy leads to vision loss from swelling in the retina, bleeding in the eye, and/or retinal detachment.

Diabetic retinopathy is the most common vascular disease to affect the eye. While age-related macular degeneration is the most common cause of visual loss in patients 60 years of age or older in the United States, diabetic retinopathy is the most common cause of visual loss in working-age patients in the United States. Diabetic retinopathy is strongly related to blood sugar control. The better the blood sugar control, the less likely patients are to develop significant retinopathy or to experience progression of current retinopathy. While age-related macular degeneration and diabetic retinopathy do not directly affect disease progress of one another, visual loss from one can certainly have a dramatic impact on patients who have already experienced visual loss from the other. Therefore,

Cotton-wool spots
Small, fluffy white patches seen on retinal examination. They are secondary to ischemia and are often seen in diabetic retinopathy.

While age-related macular degeneration is the most common cause of visual loss in patients 60 years of age or older in the United States, diabetic retinopathy is the most common cause of visual loss in working-age patients in the United States.

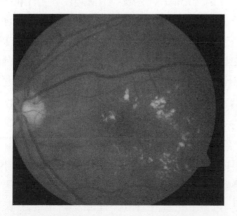

Figure 16   Diabetic retinopathy.

patients with diabetic retinopathy should do everything possible to maximize their blood sugar control, blood pressure control, and any other factors that could lead to worsening of their retinopathy.

61. What are the chances of getting wet macular degeneration in my good eye?

A general rule of thumb is that wet macular degeneration occurs roughly 50% of the time over a 5-year period in the fellow eye of a patient who has wet macular degeneration. There are certain characteristics that tell us whether patients are at somewhat increased or decreased risk of this occurring. The presence of large, soft drusen and/or significant retinal pigment epithelium (the layer underneath the retina) abnormalities suggest an increased risk of developing wet macular degeneration. The absence of any such findings and/or the presence of minimal or small drusen suggest a lesser risk. These risk factors may be modified by actions such as vitamin supplementation; therefore it is strongly recommended that all at-risk patients follow the AREDS recommendations.

62. What causes scarring of the retina?

The abnormal blood vessels that grow underneath and into the retina often lead to a scar over time. In a minority of cases, the disease is caught early enough that regression or disappearance of the vessels may occur; however, in most cases, the vessels are far enough along that even though treatment prevents them from leaking further, they do not disappear. They subsequently end up as a fibrous or thickened scar. The new vessels often release factors that signal additional cells to come to the area of wet macular degeneration. These additional cells lead to an inflammatory reaction that results in scarring. Finally, bleeding that occurs in association with wet macular degeneration in and of itself can bring about factors that can lead to scarring. Current research includes new treatments that may help to prevent scarring or that may even lead to regression, or breakdown, of scars that have already formed.

PART SIX

Treatment for Wet Macular Degeneration: New Therapies, Similarities and Differences, Risks and Benefits

How do anti-VEGF agents work?

What is the difference between Lucentis and Avastin?

What happens if I stop responding to the treatments?

More . . .

63. How do anti-VEGF agents work?

Vascular endothelial growth factor (VEGF) is a factor normally found in the eye that helps to promote new blood vessel growth. As discussed in Question 59, prior to birth VEGF is believed to play a critical role in the development of blood vessels in the eye, as well as other parts of the body. Once a person is born, the role of VEGF is less clear. While VEGF still plays a role in normal physiologic activities in the body, it is also known to play a critical role in the development of abnormal blood vessels in the body. This has been demonstrated in numerous clinical trials in which various inhibitors of VEGF have led to prevention of various disease characteristics or prevention of the disease altogether.

Anti-VEGF agents, such as Lucentis of Avastin, work by blocking VEGF. VEGF is required for the growth of the abnormal new blood vessels associated with wet macular degeneration. Anti-VEGF agents either bind to circulating VEGF, preventing it from binding to its receptor, or anti-VEGF agents may actually block the receptor, preventing circulating VEGF from attaching to the receptor. VEGF must bind with its receptor to initiate its actions, such as blood vessel growth or increased leaking. Other anti-VEGF therapies currently under investigation may try to inhibit the production of VEGF on a molecular level—that is, before it is even made. All anti-VEGF therapies share the common goal of preventing VEGF from carrying out its actions.

Lucentis treatments have demonstrated a rather remarkable ability to stabilize vision loss from wet macular degeneration.

64. Will Lucentis or Avastin injections help my vision improve?

First and foremost, Lucentis treatments have demonstrated a rather remarkable ability to stabilize vision loss from wet macular degeneration. In the important pivotal trials upon which Lucentis received FDA (Food and Drug Administration) approval for the treatment of wet macular degeneration, roughly 80% of all patients experienced true stabilization, meaning that they either did not lose any vision or they gained vision with treatment. The large majority of these patients actually experienced some degree of visual gain. Even more encouraging is the fact that 30–40% of the patients treated in these studies experienced *significant* visual gain, meaning they actually gained three lines or more on the eye chart.

Avastin did not go through pivotal eye trials as did Lucentis because Avastin was already approved for the treatment of colorectal cancer, and its use is off-label for the treatment of wet macular degeneration. Thus, more formal results for Avastin's treatment of macular degeneration are not known. However, numerous published small series and case reports of patients treated with Avastin have indicated similar results to Lucentis. Currently, a large trial comparing Avastin to Lucentis is under way.

If 80% of patients treated with these medications are stable, then 20% of patients still experience visual loss. This loss can be anywhere from mild, such as losing one or two letters on the eye chart, to significant, meaning losing three lines or more. Small numbers of patients, roughly 5–10%, experience significant visual loss. These findings do not necessarily mean that the treatments are not working, as the loss may be due to something other than wet macular degeneration, such as dry macular degeneration, glaucoma, or cataract. For instance, even though the wet macular degeneration may be under control from the treatments, patients may still experience visual loss due to underlying dry macular degeneration that is not treated with the injections.

65. What is the difference between Lucentis and Avastin?

Lucentis is a drug that was designed to treat wet macular degeneration by injection into the eye. Scientists and researchers determined the characteristics that would make an intraocular medication most effective and molded Lucentis in this manner. Avastin's active component is similar to the active component in Lucentis. However, Avastin was not designed as an eye treatment but rather as an anticancer medicine. Its recommended path of administration is by intravenous infusion, and it was approved by the FDA for the treatment of metastatic colorectal cancer in 2004. It has subsequently been shown that it is also effective in the treatment of metastatic breast cancer and small cell lung cancer.

A major difference between Avastin and Lucentis is the size of the agents. Avastin is a full-length antibody, which gives it a certain degree of lasting power when administered intravenously. Lucentis is what is known as an antibody fragment (i.e., it is a fragment of a full-length antibody), and therefore it is a smaller drug that was believed to confer certain properties, such as better penetration into the retina when injected into the eye. These differences are theoretical, and whether or not they manifest as actual treatment differences remains to be determined. Small studies have suggested a potential advantage to Lucentis with regard to initial treatment benefit and an advantage to Avastin with regard to treatment duration. However, these studies are not definitive, and a large national randomized trial is currently being conducted to help answer questions regarding the benefits of Lucentis and Avastin relative to one another.

66. Why is Avastin so much cheaper than Lucentis? Does this mean it is not as good a drug?

Avastin is roughly 1/40 (2.5%) the cost of Lucentis per intraocular injection ($50 as compared to $2000). This cost difference is in no way related to the effectiveness of the drugs. It is important to remember that the costs were determined at the time of initial approval of each drug. When Avastin was approved by the FDA, it was done so as an anticancer drug. It was administered intravenously and required a relatively large amount (when compared to the small amount used in intraocular injections), and the cost was for this intravenous application. The price of Lucentis was determined based on the amount needed for an intraocular injection and was the price for a much smaller amount of medication. When clinicians determined that Avastin could also be injected into the eye, pharmacies would prepare intraocular injections by taking a single intravenous anticancer dose and dividing it up into multiple intraocular doses. This method resulted in the much higher priced oncology dose being divided into a number of intraocular doses, which ultimately resulted in a significantly less expensive per-dose amount.

67. Why are treatments for wet macular degeneration often derived from cancer therapies?

Cancer and wet macular degeneration have characteristics in common. Cancer is best thought of as an abnormal growth of cells that are not responsive to normal mechanisms of inhibition. In the body, some cells grow or replenish as certain cells die off. This process is necessary for maintenance of normal body functions. Cancer occurs when cells grow in an abnormal or pathologic fashion and are not receptive to normal feedback mechanisms. Wet macular degeneration is an abnormal or unbridled growth of blood vessels that would not occur in a normal setting.

One strategy for treating cancers is to use agents that shut down the blood vessels that supply the cancer. These agents are termed **antiangiogenic agents** and are believed to work by essentially starving the tumors (i.e., the blood vessels bring nutrition and other factors necessary for growth to the tumors). Similarly, antiangiogenic agents are highly effective therapies against wet macular degeneration by shutting down these abnormal blood vessels. Another treatment, **photodynamic therapy**, involves the use of a photosensitizing dye and a **cold laser** (or subthreshold laser). This treatment also began as a cancer therapy and was later found to be effective as a treatment for wet macular degeneration.

68. What percentage of patients respond well to Lucentis?

The large majority of patients respond well to Lucentis. A response can be measured in several ways. In the large pivotal studies that led to Lucentis being approved by the FDA, the major outcome that was measured was prevention of moderate vision loss. This meant that patients lost less than 15 letters on the eye chart. This finding may seem like a rather negative response for prevention as opposed to gaining letters, but it is important to realize that prior to the approval of Lucentis, all treatments for wet macular degeneration were measured by their ability to prevent 15-letter loss. It was very unusual for any treatments to truly stabilize patients—i.e., prevent any loss; therefore,

Antiangiogenic agents

Drugs that prevent the growth of new blood vessels. Avastin and Lucentis are examples of such agents.

Photodynamic therapy

An approved therapy for wet macular degeneration in which a photosensitizing dye is injected into a patient's arm, and a cold or low-energy laser is used to treat the new blood vessels.

Cold laser

A laser that works through the use of low power or intensity. With regard to macular degeneration, this refers to the use of photodynamic therapy, a laser that acts on abnormal vessels that have been activated by a photosensitizing dye (verteporfin).

treatments were measured by their ability to limit or slow vision loss. Most treatments prevented 50–60% of patients from losing 15 letters over a 1- to 2-year duration. Lucentis, however, prevented approximately 90% of patients from losing 15 letters over a 2-year span. Moreover, the ability of Lucentis to treat patients effectively went well beyond these measurements. Approximately 80% of patients who were treated with Lucentis were truly stable—i.e., lost no letters of vision or actually gained vision. Roughly one-third of all patients treated actually gained 15 letters of visual acuity. Previous treatments led to 2–6% of all patients gaining this degree of vision. These outcomes have truly changed patients' and physicians' approach and expectations with regard to wet macular degeneration.

69. What percentage of patients respond well to Avastin?

The actual percentage of patients responding well to Avastin is not fully known. Lucentis was the focus of several large randomized clinical trials. Randomized clinical trials are the most definitive means of evaluating a treatment. As Lucentis results began to be reported at scientific meetings, retina specialists started using Avastin for the treatment of wet macular degeneration. They recognized that Avastin and Lucentis treat new blood vessels similarly, and they began to test Avastin first systemically (administered by intravenous therapy) and then via an intraocular injection. It became clear that Avastin was also highly effective for the treatment of wet macular degeneration, and its use was quickly adopted by retina specialists across the United States and then elsewhere.

While its efficacy was clearly appreciated, actual scientific evaluation via randomized clinical trials was not available (see Question 64); therefore, it is not known if Avastin is as effective or as safe as Lucentis, although accumulation of available data suggests they are comparable. Presently, a large clinical trial (**CATT**) is enrolling patients to compare Avastin to Lucentis. One must keep in mind that while Avastin has been widely adapted and appears to be a relatively safe and effective drug, its use is still off-label, and less is known about the effects of Avastin relative to Lucentis.

CATT

Comparison of Age-Related Macular Degeneration Treatment Trial, a multicenter, randomized treatment trial evaluating the relative safety and efficacy of Lucentis versus Avastin.

70. Are Avastin and Lucentis the only anti-VEGF treatments used in wet macular degeneration?

Avastin and Lucentis are not the only anti-VEGF treatments used for wet macular degeneration. In fact, the very first anti-VEGF therapy approved for the treatment of macular degeneration was **Macugen** (pegaptanib). Macugen was approved in December of 2004, prior to the approval of Lucentis, for all types of wet macular degeneration; however, the efficacy of Macugen was not nearly as robust as that of Lucentis. Clinical trials showed that while Macugen slowed vision loss in the majority of patients, patients were relatively unlikely to experience significant visual improvement. Roughly 6% of patients in the study improved significantly versus roughly 33% of patients treated with Lucentis. In addition, patients were far more likely to stabilize with Lucentis than they were with Macugen. With the approval of Lucentis and with the rapid adoption of Avastin, Macugen's use dropped dramatically.

Macugen

An approved anti-VEGF agent that is used in the treatment of wet macular degeneration.

71. I am not experiencing any vision loss now, but my retina specialist is recommending treatment for my recently diagnosed wet macular degeneration. Do I need to have treatment right away?

Wet age-related macular degeneration is often diagnosed when visual loss has occurred. Patients will notice distorted or blurred vision and go to see their eye care provider. Once diagnosed, treatment with an anti-VEGF agent such as Lucentis or Avastin is often initiated. While these agents are excellent at preventing further vision loss, and even lead to visual gain in a significant percentage of patients, the visual prognosis is typically related to the initial vision. Therefore, if patients are fortunate enough to have minimal vision loss at the time of diagnosis, their overall prognosis is much better, especially if treatment can be initiated prior to visual loss. While it has not been absolutely demonstrated in clinical trials, if the current therapies have an 80% chance of preventing any vision loss, and patients initiate therapy without significant visual loss, then there is an excellent chance that the therapy will maintain their current level of vision. For this reason, when wet macular degeneration is diagnosed, regardless of whether there has been visual loss, treatment should be initiated as soon as possible.

When wet macular degeneration is diagnosed, regardless of whether there has been visual loss, treatment should be initiated as soon as possible.

Nick's comment:

I credit my understanding of the sense of urgency of this disease to my eye doctor, who asked if I could go in to see a specialist THAT DAY! Since then I have learned more about how important it is to respond quickly to any changes in vision. Even today, I will travel, but I will not go more than a day's flight away from my doctor.

72. I developed wet macular degeneration several years ago and was very excited to learn about the new treatments for it; however, when I contacted my doctor, he informed me that it was unlikely that these treatments would help me. Why is this so?

The new treatments for wet macular degeneration, in particular the anti-VEGF injections, are directed toward stopping the new blood vessels from forming and preventing the leakage associated with new blood vessels of recent onset. Recent onset means days to weeks and, in some cases, even months. These new treatments are unlikely to make a significant difference if the wet macular degeneration has been present for a long period of time (i.e., years). Over time, scarring and degeneration of retinal tissues takes place secondary to wet macular degeneration, and irreversible changes occur in the retina. These changes are usually not impacted by current macular degeneration treatments and therefore the vision loss cannot be reversed.

Subretinal

Beneath the retina.

Intraretinal

Occurring within the retina, such as a hemorrhage or swelling.

However, there are some cases in which the current treatments can make a difference. Despite longstanding disease of even several years, some patients have **subretinal** and **intraretinal** fluid associated with their wet macular degeneration, often with active leakage present. In such cases, a trial of one or a few Lucentis or Avastin injections may be performed to see if the leakage can be stopped and vision improved. It is reasonable to contact your retina specialist to ensure that he or she does not believe you will benefit from such therapy.

73. Will insurance cover my macular degeneration treatments?

Lucentis was approved by the FDA for the treatment of wet macular degeneration in the summer of 2006. Following that approval, the majority of insurance companies, including Medicare, have accepted it as the standard of care for treating wet macular degeneration. Due to the significant cost of this treatment, it is always recommended that patients check with their insurance companies, both their primary and their secondary, if they have one, to ensure that it is covered. If patients have only a primary insurance with a co-pay, it is recommended that they inquire about the co-pay ahead of time, as the co-pay alone can be quite significant. They may be eligible for programs by Genentech, the manufacturer of Lucentis, that would help to cover the co-pay. Avastin was approved by the FDA for the treatment of colorectal cancer; however, due to its relatively low cost, many—if not most—insurance plans will cover it for the treatment of wet macular degeneration. Again, it is recommended that patients check with their individual plans to ensure that this is the case. In the event that an insurance company does not cover a patient's treatments, it is recommended that the patient contact Genentech to see if they have a program that would help pay for treatments.

74. If I don't have insurance, how can I possibly afford to pay for treatments of wet macular degeneration?

Patients without health coverage should contact Genentech directly and inquire about their programs for helping patients, such as those without insurance, get coverage. Programs do exist for just this type of situation, and experts at Genentech will help you to determine whether you are eligible for their programs (http://www.gene.com). Some patients have primary insurance but no secondary insurance to help with co-pays. Co-pays are typically around 20% of the overall cost, and can be quite expensive when treating with Lucentis. The choice of anti-VEGF treatment, Lucentis or Avastin, is often determined by the retina specialist based upon various criteria including the specialist's comfort level with one drug or the other. In cases where insurance or the co-pay is an issue, the retina specialist will often initiate treatment with Avastin, but switch to Lucentis if the result is less than that expected.

75. Does wet macular degeneration recur? If so, how often?

In many patients, if not most, with wet macular degeneration, active leaking stops after receiving a series of Lucentis or Avastin injections. In addition, the fluid that was leaking becomes reabsorbed. At this point, your physician, in consultation with you, may elect to follow your condition without additional treatments or to space your treatments at certain intervals. While a percentage of patients do not develop recurrences, the majority of patients do have recurrent episodes of leakage. Roughly 80% or greater of all patients develop recurrences within the first year. This high percentage should not be viewed as a failure of the therapy. Recurrences are relatively common and typically respond to additional therapy. Recurrent leakage may occur within 1 to 2 months of stopping therapy, although it is not uncommon for it to recur several months later. Some patients develop recurrences with regular frequency, possibly every 2 to 3 months, or as infrequently as every 6 months or longer. Therefore, it is important once therapy has been put on hold for patients to monitor

While a percentage of patients do not develop recurrences, the majority of patients do have recurrent episodes of leakage.

their vision carefully and to continue with regular follow-up visits with their retina specialist.

Some retina specialists prefer to continue therapy on a monthly or relatively frequent regimen. Monthly injections were performed in the pivotal trials that led to the FDA's approval of Lucentis. Smaller studies have demonstrated good results using Lucentis or Avastin on an as-needed basis. The potential benefits and risks of monthly therapy versus treatment on an as-needed basis are also being studied in the same trial that is looking at the efficacy of Lucentis versus Avastin (CATT).

76. What happens if I stop responding to the treatments?

While it is uncommon for patients to stop responding to the intraocular injections, it does happen in a small percentage of patients. When this occurs, the retina specialist may consider using combination therapy, which typically involves the use of photodynamic therapy and anti-VEGF injections. It may also include the use of a **steroid** injection.

Photodynamic therapy involves intravenous infusion of a photosensitizing drug into a patient's arm. The drug is taken up by the abnormal blood vessels in the eye, and these vessels are then sensitized to what is referred to as a cold, or subthreshold, laser. Cold lasers operate at a power that theoretically does not affect normal vessels or normal tissues, but is absorbed by the abnormal vessels (those that have taken up the dye). Photodynamic therapy was approved for the treatment of wet macular degeneration in the year 2000, but it was only believed to be effective for a small percentage of patients (those with a particular type of wet macular degeneration, determined by fluorescein angiography). In addition, it was found most

Steroids

Anti-inflammatory agents used to treat a variety of medical conditions. They may be administered systemically (intravenously or orally), by injection, or topically.

effective as a means of slowing vision loss, but not preventing it or helping to restore vision. Recent studies have suggested that photodynamic therapy is far more effective when used in combination with anti-VEGF injections, and it may be useful for patients with new-onset wet macular degeneration as well as those with more refractory lesions. In addition, new approaches to wet macular degeneration are currently being evaluated and offer the potential of alternative therapies to those patients who experience suboptimal responses to current therapy.

77. What happens if I elect not to have treatment for exudative macular degeneration? What happens if I elect to discontinue therapy for wet macular degeneration?

Therapy for wet macular degeneration is aimed at stabilizing and/or improving vision. As discussed in other questions, these treatments are extremely effective at stabilizing vision, and a significant number of patients have visual improvement. Numerous studies have shown us that without therapy, patients with wet macular degeneration experience vision loss over a one-to-two-year span. This is the result of ongoing leakage, bleeding, and ultimately scarring. In most patients, this process stabilizes with time so that an end-stage or advanced stage is reached where little additional vision loss occurs. This stage varies from individual to individual. Some patients with wet macular degeneration experience little vision loss without treatment. The majority, however, do lose vision, typically to the point of becoming legally blind (20/200 or worse) in the eye with wet macular degeneration. In the large majority of cases peripheral vision is unaffected, and therefore withholding or refusing treatment for exudative macular degeneration usually only affects central vision.

If patients are currently undergoing therapy and elect to discontinue therapy, their course is largely dependent on the stage of their disease. If they have received a number of treatments and the exudative or wet stage of the disease has stabilized, it is possible that they will not experience further vision loss; however in many, if not most, patients, the therapy is the reason for stabilization of the disease and at some point after discontinuing therapy, a recurrence or flare-up of the wet macular degeneration may occur, resulting in further vision loss.

78. I have heard that patients with a history of stroke or cardiac disease should not get the injections. Can the injection cause a stroke or heart attack?

It is unlikely that the anti-VEGF injections, such as Lucentis or Avastin, cause strokes or heart attacks in patients, with the possible exception of patients who have suffered recent strokes or heart attacks—specifically, within the previous 6 to 12 months. Large clinical studies did not reveal clinically significant risks, meaning a risk of stroke or heart attack that was clearly due to anti-VEGF injections in patients other than those who experienced recent vascular events, such as stroke or heart attack. As more and more patients are being treated, clinicians and the companies that make these treatments are following this concern carefully to ensure patient safety. Patients with a significant vascular or cardiac history should consult their primary care physician when wet macular degeneration is diagnosed and treatment with either Lucentis or Avastin is recommended. If patients about to undergo treatment have any concerns or questions regarding their safety, they should talk with both their medical and eye care doctors.

PART SEVEN

Intravitreal Injections: How Are They Given, Do They Hurt, and What Should I Worry About?

How many injections will I need?

Do the injections hurt?

What should I expect to see after the injections?

More . . .

79. How are the injections administered?

Injections are typically administered right in your doctor's office (they are occasionally administered in a procedure room or operating room). Patients are placed in an exam chair, which is often tilted back to allow the head to rest. Topical anesthetic drops are placed on the eye. Several drops of **Betadine** (an antiseptic solution) are placed on the eye as well. The lids and surrounding skin of the eye are treated with a Betadine prep. A sterile drape may or may not be placed over the treated eye. Your retina specialist will then anesthetize the eye either with a topical anesthetic or a **subconjunctival** anesthetic. The subconjunctival anesthetic is administered by a very fine needle in the layer just overlying the white part of the eye. When the eye is anesthetized (which typically only takes around a minute or so), a **lid speculum** is placed into the eye to hold the lids and lashes back from the injection site. Alternatively, many doctors reproduce the actions of a lid speculum by holding the lids apart or having their assistant hold the lids. Another drop of Betadine is placed over the injection site. The retina specialist will then inject the medication using a small syringe with a very fine needle. The injection itself takes a matter of a few seconds. The injecting physician may or may not use a Q-tip to apply pressure lightly to the injection site. An antibiotic drop is then often placed on the injection site, and the lid speculum is removed.

Betadine

A povidone-iodine scrub used prior to surgery or other form of medical treatment to disinfect the area to be treated.

Subconjunctival

Under the thin transparent covering of the white part of the eye.

Lid speculum

A piece of equipment that holds the eye open and the lids out of the way during procedures such as cataract surgery or intravitreal injections.

80. How many injections will I need?

The number of injections each patient needs is based on his or her individual situation. The original studies, which demonstrated the benefit of these treatments, required that patients be treated monthly for up to 2 years. Another study showed that patients who received three initial injections spaced monthly and were then treated quarterly (every 3 months) demonstrated a benefit, but the benefit was not as robust as those patients who were treated monthly. Current treatment regimens vary from physician to physician. Most patients receive somewhere between one to four injections spaced monthly, and are then monitored with various follow-up plans, with follow-ups ranging anywhere from monthly to quarterly.

Apart from monthly therapy, which is relatively uncommon at present, two regimens are commonly used. In the first, patients receive three to four injections and are then followed at various intervals and retreated only if recurrent leakage is noted. In a second plan, patients receive three to four injections and then have their follow-up visits extended with each visit, with injections at each follow-up. For instance, if they are seen after 1 month and not noted to have any leakage, they are treated at that time and their next follow-up may be set for 6 weeks. If they come back in 6 weeks and are not noted to have any leakage, they are given an injection at that time, with their next follow-up set at 2 months. These periods are rarely extended beyond 3 months. A third, less common, regimen is that followed in the pivotal studies resulting in the approval of Lucentis by the FDA—treatment monthly regardless of resolution of fluid or recurrence of new blood vessels.

Patients often elect one of the first two regimens rather than the third due to the burden of frequent injections and visits both for the patient and for his or her family. Decisions such as these should include patients, their retina specialist, and their family. Ongoing studies may help to further clarify the best regimen. It is still important that patients undergo routine follow-up and that they understand that each case is different and that their doctor will help to determine what is best for them. Studies are currently being conducted to help retina specialists determine the best treatment regimens.

81. Do the injections hurt?

Intraocular injections are easily tolerated by patients, with little to no pain noted.

Intraocular injections are easily tolerated by patients, with little to no pain noted. The eye is numbed prior to the injection with either topical or subconjunctival anesthetic. Patients may notice pressure or an occasional mild to moderate amount of pain that quickly resolves after the injection. Most patients do not require any type of pain medication following the injection. For those who do, usually acetaminophen or ibuprofen suffices. Occasionally, patients notice pain after the anesthetic wears off. This pain is usually mild. In the infrequent instances when significant pain is noted, it is usually due to a corneal abrasion (an inadvertent scratch of the cornea). Topical ointment helps to alleviate the pain, and the abrasion usually heals overnight. Keeping the eyes closed and resting may also help to reduce the discomfort. If pain is not relieved with these steps and an over-the-counter oral pain medicine, the patient should contact his or her retina specialist.

Nick's comment:

I found the injection procedures to be reasonably painless and soon realized that my concerns were mostly in my head. I learned to focus on how fortunate I was to be getting the treatment. I had once seen a blind teenage girl who was walking with a red and white cane. I frequently recalled this vision and contrasted it to the opportunity that I had with Lucentis.

82. Can I see the needle coming toward my eye?

In most cases, your retina specialist will approach your eye from the direction opposite which you are looking. You are usually aware of the approach, but not of the needle. You will not be able to close your fellow eye, as that would make your treated eye turn up and out. Your retina specialist will direct your eye to allow the injection to be administered in certain positions. It is certainly reasonable to discuss your concerns with your retina specialist prior to the injection.

83. Should I stop taking aspirin before the injection?

There is no need to discontinue aspirin prior to or during a course of injections. Bleeding inside the eye is a very uncommon complication of the injection and rarely requires any type of treatment. Bleeding on the outside or white part of the eye occasionally occurs, but it is usually mild and self-limited. It can be more common following a certain type of anesthesia, called subconjunctival anesthesia, which involves an injection underneath the thin covering of the white part of the eye. This injection occasionally can hit or touch small, barely visible vessels, causing a small hemorrhage. These hemorrhages are visually insignificant and typically clear within a week or two. While they may look disconcerting, they are of little concern. These hemorrhages are far less common with topical anesthesia. Aspirin doesn't cause these hemorrhages, but it can make them a little worse if they occur.

84. What should I expect to see after the injections?

Immediately following the injection, a veil or clumping of gel-like material can be visualized. This is occasionally accompanied by small black spots, or **floaters**. Less commonly, a small to somewhat larger black circle can be seen, often representing small air bubbles that are present in the syringe at the time of injection. These side effects are harmless and will resolve within a day or two. If you notice a new shower of floaters, short flashing lights, or an opaque shade or curtain, then call your retina specialist. This development will most likely result in a relatively quick return to the office and repeat retinal examination. While these symptoms (the flashing lights and the floaters) are often benign, there is a risk of retinal tear and/or detachment; patients with such symptoms should be checked carefully. If different symptoms occur, or if you become concerned about some component of the post-injection course, contact your retina specialist.

Floaters

Spots of various size and shape within the eye, seen within a person's visual field. They may be inflammatory cells, pigment cells from tears in the retina, or small air bubbles from an intraocular injection.

85. What precautions should I follow after an injection?

Patients should be aware of the risk of an infection and should avoid activities that could increase this risk. For example, in the next several days, they should avoid swimming in a pool or hot tub. The risk of infection, however, is very low. Patients should be certain to report any increases in redness or pain, or decreases in vision, in the several days following an injection. If there is any question of these symptoms occurring, or if additional concerns exist, patients should contact their retina specialist immediately.

Patients should be certain to report any increases in redness or pain, or decreases in vision, in the several days following an injection.

86. I'm afraid of getting injections in the eye. Is there a pill I can take instead?

Although oral medications have been studied for wet macular degeneration, no oral treatment has demonstrated efficacy to date. One of the biggest problems with oral treatments is the need to take a large amount of medication to allow delivery of an appropriate amount to the eye. When a sufficient amount is taken, treatment is often complicated by systemic side effects. For instance, when Avastin was first used to treat wet macular degeneration, it was administered via infusion into blood vessels in the arm (as it is used for the treatment of cancer). Although this effectively treated the new vessels in the eyes, it also led to significant side effects, the most frequent of which was increased blood pressure. Therefore, it was further tested via intraocular injection and demonstrated clinical success and minimal systemic side effects. Clinical trials are evaluating various non-injection approaches, including other oral medications and topical administration. However, intraocular injections remain the only approved and clinically proven treatment for wet macular degeneration.

Intravitreal Injections

PART EIGHT

Other Treatments: Cold Lasers, Combination Therapies, Future Possibilities

What do I do if my wet macular degeneration does not respond to normal therapy?

I often hear of research trials described in phases, such as phase I, II, III, or IV. What do the different phases mean, and how do they apply to clinical research?

Are there natural therapies for treating age-related macular degeneration?

More . . .

87. Are there therapies other than anti-VEGF therapy that are approved for the treatment of wet macular degeneration?

Anti-VEGF therapies are a relatively recent addition to treatments used for wet macular degeneration. The first anti-VEGF therapy, Macugen, was approved in 2004. Lucentis was approved in June of 2006. Avastin was approved in 2004 for the treatment of colorectal cancer, and its use for wet macular degeneration began in the summer of 2005 as an off-label therapy. Prior to anti-VEGF therapies, two different lasers had been approved for the treatment of wet macular degeneration. Conventional laser, or laser that uses heat or energy to shut down or prevent the growth of abnormal tissues, was studied and approved as therapy for wet macular degeneration in the 1980s. Unfortunately, tissues adjacent to those treated were also affected. As a result, abnormal vessels were often shut down, but vision was lost or visual gain was typically unattainable due to the laser. Despite tissue damage, long-term studies showed that many patients still benefited from laser because over several years, less damage ultimately occurred from laser than from the natural progression of wet macular degeneration. In other words, the acute visual loss associated with laser was often less than the long-term visual loss associated with wet macular degeneration.

More recently, a different type of laser, photodynamic therapy, was approved for treatment of certain patients with wet macular degeneration. Photodynamic therapy (see Question 76) utilizes a photosensitizing dye and a cold, or subthreshold, laser. The theoretical advantage of photodynamic therapy is that it allows for destruction of abnormal blood vessels without damage to adjacent tissues. Unfortunately, most patients with wet macular degeneration are not good candidates for photodynamic therapy based on the characteristics of their wet macular degeneration. With the introduction of anti-VEGF agents, photodynamic therapy has been used less frequently; however, a resurgence of use has occurred over the past couple years as photodynamic therapy has demonstrated some degree of efficacy in combination therapy with intraocular anti-VEGF therapies, as well as with **intravitreal** steroids.

88. Is there ever a role for laser in the treatment of wet macular degeneration?

There are some cases of wet macular degeneration that may be amenable to conventional laser. Patients who develop small, well-defined areas of new blood vessel growth that are far removed from the center of vision may be good candidates for laser treatment. Laser to these noncentral areas of vessel growth do not typically result in damage to central vision. Although a scotoma, or blind spot, occurs at the site of the laser, it often does not bother patients if it is far removed from the central retina. The benefit of laser in such situations is that a single treatment may be all that is needed, obviating the need for repeat treatments. Studies have shown that patients who are treated with laser have a roughly 50% chance of recurrences. In the event of recurrences, the vessel growth is frequently closer to the center of vision; therefore these patients must be followed regularly, and administration of intraocular injections with anti-VEGF therapy is frequently necessary.

Intravitreal

Into the vitreous cavity, the posterior compartment of the eye (which is occupied by a gel-like material called the vitreous). Lucentis or Avastin therapy is administered by injection into the vitreous cavity.

Patients who develop small, well-defined areas of new blood vessel growth that are far removed from the center of vision may be good candidates for laser treatment.

Other Treatments

89. What do I do if my wet macular degeneration does not respond to normal therapy?

The large majority of patients with wet macular degeneration respond to anti-VEGF injections. Eighty percent of patients show absolutely no further loss and/or visual gain. More than 90% of patients show only minimal loss or a gain in vision. The majority of patients show resolution of fluid that has leaked from wet macular degeneration; however, there is a small percentage of patients who do not respond to these treatments. This failure to respond may be due to variants of wet macular degeneration that are somewhat less responsive to these treatments. In these cases, your retina specialist may talk to you about the benefits of combination therapy. Recent reports suggest some benefit of photodynamic therapy, anti-VEGF injection, and intravitreal steroid injection (see Question 76). This treatment may be beneficial in patients with new-onset disease as well as those whose disease did not respond initially. Ongoing clinical trials will hopefully answer these questions.

90. Are therapies ever combined in the treatment of wet macular degeneration?

Therapies may be combined when treating wet macular degeneration. An early combination therapy occurred when photodynamic therapy and intraocular steroids were used together. Small studies showed that the combination of these two agents both lengthened the duration of treatment and increased the apparent efficacy of either treatment alone. However, with the introduction of anti-VEGF agents, this combination was used less frequently. More recently, small studies have demonstrated the efficacy of photodynamic therapy, anti-VEGF agents, and occasional intraocular steroid use in the treatment of wet macular degeneration (see Question 76). This combination is often referred to as triple therapy, and, at least in smaller studies, it has demonstrated efficacy similar to anti-VEGF agents alone, but with a greater duration of treatment effect. Triple therapy is currently the focus of several larger clinical trials.

A few clinicians have even evaluated a "quadruple" therapy approach, which combines photodynamic therapy, anti-VEGF agents, intravitreal steroids, and a vitrectomy (a surgical procedure in which the vitreous, the gel in the back of the eye, is removed). Further studies are necessary to determine the relative benefits of each of these combinations.

91. Steroids are used to treat so many medical conditions. Can they be used for age-related macular degeneration?

Steroids have many unique properties that make them important in the treatment of medical conditions. In general, they are used to treat conditions that are related to inflammation, such as autoimmune diseases and asthma. Steroids have been tried in various manners for the treatment of wet macular degeneration. As monotherapy (used as the only treatment), the results have been disappointing. There is some effect, but it is not very effective, however, steroids have been used in combination with other treatments with some degree of success. As mentioned previously, they have been used in combination with photodynamic therapy. The initial results were somewhat promising, with some patients experiencing stabilization or improvement in vision. Subsequent studies also demonstrated a treatment benefit, but not as robust as the initial reports. This treatment became less useful with the introduction of anti-VEGF therapy. A more recent approach has been the combination of anti-VEGF therapy, photodynamic therapy, and steroids, a combination referred to as triple therapy. Further study is warranted to determine whether this treatment actually offers benefit over currently accepted anti-VEGF therapy. In all of these approaches, the steroids are administered by an intraocular injection, allowing for delivery of the steroid to the area where it is needed without significant systemic absorption.

The biggest concern regarding steroid use is the risk of complications, both systemic and ocular. Systemic complications of steroid use include difficulty sleeping, weight gain, and psychological effects, such as increased or decreased energy and/or mood swings. The concern over systemic side effects virtually eliminates systemic use (either orally or by intravenous administration) in the treatment of macular degeneration. Ocular complications include increased intraocular pressure and cataracts. (Once cataracts are removed, there is no risk of them recurring, whether steroids are used or not.) The ocular complications, especially the risk of increased intraocular pressure, limit the use of steroids in patients who are at high risk of developing glaucoma, or those who already have glaucoma.

92. Considering that many cancer therapies have led to macular degeneration treatments, can radiation therapy be used for macular degeneration?

Radiation therapy has been used in previous studies for wet macular degeneration with varying degrees of success. While it has demonstrated biologic activity, meaning it has been shown to affect the growth of new blood vessels from wet macular degeneration, the challenge has been to deliver the radiation with minimal side effects. Radiation is known to have characteristics that are beneficial in the treatment of wet macular degeneration. It is strongly antiangiogenic (prevents new blood vessel growth), **antifibrotic** (inhibits scarring), and **anti-inflammatory** (inhibits inflammation), all characteristics that would be helpful in the treatment of this disease. In addition, radiation therapy is known to demonstrate synergism with other treatment modalities, meaning it has beneficial effects in combination with other treatments. For example, in the treatment of colorectal cancer, radiation therapy has been used in combination with Avastin. As a result, several companies are actively looking at its potential role in the treatment of wet macular degeneration.

One treatment approach utilizes a device that delivers the radiation therapy via surgery directly to the area of wet macular degeneration. This approach allows a significant dose of radiation to be delivered directly to the affected area, with minimal effects on the surrounding tissues. The radioactive isotope that is used, **strontium-90**, has a biologic effect that falls off rapidly as a function of distance from the source of delivery. In the past, radiation therapy has been of concern in the eye because of damage to the retina, optic nerve, and lens; however, preliminary studies with this approach have not revealed damage to these tissues. Further evaluation is necessary and is ongoing, as many of these effects may occur several years after application. Initial study results in which Avastin and this radiation approach were combined were encouraging, with stabilization of vision and vision gains similar to those with Avastin or Lucentis. In addition, patients were treated infrequently, with relatively few additional injections other

Antifibrotic

A drug or treatment that prevents or limits fibrosis (scarring).

Anti-inflammatory

A drug or treatment that prevents or inhibits inflammation.

Strontium-90

Strontium-90 is a radioactive source used in the treatment of some cancers. It is also currently being studied in the treatment of wet macular degeneration.

than the initial two mandated by the study. Potential issues with this approach include the risks of incurring a surgical procedure (potential complications include cataract, bleeding, infection, and retinal detachment) and the probable limitation of only being able to deliver the radiation treatment once.

In a second approach, low-energy x-rays with minimal scatter are administered via a device that fits easily in an office (the device is similar to those seen in a dental office). This device utilizes robotic control of the eye position, allowing precise treatment to be delivered via three beams that pass through the lower white part of the eye and focus on the macula. The beams are delivered one at a time. Initial results of this procedure are promising as well. However, similar to the radiation procedure, additional evaluation is necessary prior to the approval of this treatment.

93. I know that Lucentis was discovered through an extensive research program. Is there ongoing research with regard to macular degeneration?

There is extensive research addressing virtually every aspect of macular degeneration. This research includes the causes of macular degeneration, such as nutritional, environmental, and hereditary factors, the progression of macular degeneration, and the treatment of both dry and wet macular degeneration. Hundreds of millions of dollars are spent annually, and untold hours of work are put in by scientists and clinicians in the hopes of progressing our understanding of this common disease and our ability to treat it. It was efforts such as these that led to the discovery and subsequent approval of Lucentis.

Until recently (meaning the past several years), there was little research related to dry macular degeneration. Much of the work related to understanding the nutritional risk factors for developing macular degeneration, the benefits of vitamin supplementation, and the hereditary components of macular degeneration. Fortunately, that lack of research has changed dramatically. Several factors have combined to lead to the significant increase in interest in dry macular degeneration. The discovery by several independent clinics of the complement factor H gene's role in drusen has led to the realization that genetics play an important role in many, if not most, patients with macular degeneration. Genetic variations and their relationship to developing macular degeneration, patients' responses to various treatments based on these variations, and the potential of modifying disease progression or treatment response as a function of these variations are a major focus of more than 10 different companies and even more academic institutions. The recognition and understanding by researchers of the potential of neuroprotection (the ability to protect cells from dying due to various degenerative processes, as happens in dry macular degeneration) has led to numerous strategies and clinical trials aimed at preventing the progression of more advanced stages of dry macular degeneration. Breakthroughs in the understanding of the toxic effects of breakdown products in the retina, and the eye's decreasing ability to take care of them as we age, have led to additional approaches (meaning new studies with potential for stopping the progression of dry macular degeneration, perhaps at earlier stages).

The dramatic breakthrough in treatment heralded by the FDA approval of Lucentis has not discouraged others from continuing to explore new treatment approaches for wet macular degeneration (as many were afraid it would). Despite the outstanding results of Lucentis, and the frequent use of Avastin, researchers are continuing to work on new anti-VEGF agents. In addition, researchers are studying different approaches to wet macular degeneration that block or modify factors other than vascular endothelial growth factor (VEGF) that are believed to play a role in pathologic blood vessel growth. New treatments that may help to prevent scarring in the retina, or even lead to breakdown or regression of already formed abnormal blood vessels, are under development and evaluation.

The concept of combining therapies, similar to the approach that oncologists take in treating various cancers, is being heavily investigated. For instance, the benefit of using an anti-VEGF agent such as Lucentis or Avastin to immediately shut down the stimulus for new vessel growth, then following this up with an antifibrotic (antiscarring) agent, would seem to offer an ideal method of not only treating the initial visual effects of wet macular degeneration but also the more long-term effects brought on by the scarring that is often seen as the blood vessels mature and contract, distorting the retina.

Finally, research is ongoing for extended delivery devices or applications to help administer currently approved therapies in such a manner that frequent treatments would be unnecessary. For example, Lucentis or Avastin may be injected in a type of capsule that would allow slow release of the medication over a period of months, if not longer, thus alleviating the need for frequent injections. Researchers are careful, however, to recognize that it may not be in patients' best interest to receive this type of ongoing treatment, and there may actually be a benefit to having frequent treatments rather than administering the drug chronically.

94. I often hear of research trials described in phases, such as phase I, II, III, or IV. What do the different phases mean, and how do they apply to clinical research?

The phases of research refer to different points of development of a treatment approach. All medical treatments must go through required levels of testing, looking at safety and efficacy, prior to receiving approval by the FDA.

Phase I trials represent the first testing in human subjects. Phase I studies are safety and tolerability studies, the main purpose of which is to demonstrate safety of the drug or treatment when applied to humans. These trials are often performed in a small group of volunteers, often in healthy volunteers. There are some instances in which real patients are used, such as those with end-stage (or far-advanced) disease. When systemic exposure is possible or likely, these trials may be conducted in an inpatient setting, allowing monitoring of the subjects. Volunteers are often compensated for this type of study with an inconvenience fee for their time spent in the inpatient facility. Often, there is also some degree of effect studied, but the main purpose is safety. Phase I studies may address questions regarding dosing.

Phase II studies are designed to determine how well a drug works, while still collecting safety data. These studies often involve more patients than in phase I trials, including up to several hundred patients. By starting at very low doses and increasing up to the highest tolerated doses, phase II studies often help to determine different dose ranges or dosing regimens for a new treatment, expanding upon the information first addressed in phase I. Dosing regimens may also be evaluated by changing the dosing frequency throughout the course of the study. Most drugs fail in phase II testing, when a treatment effect, or absence thereof, is often detected. Data are taken from phase I and phase II studies to create phase III studies.

Phase III trials are often pivotal studies, or studies that are designed to give the final answer as to whether a new drug or treatment is worthy of use in humans—and FDA (or other country's regulatory agency) approval. Phase III trials are randomized (meaning patients are randomly assigned to different treatment groups), controlled (meaning the new treatment is compared to some other standard therapy, usually the standard of care), and multicenter. Standard of care may be simply observation, or it may be therapy with another treatment approach or pharmacologic agent. When the standard of care is observation only, the control arm is often a placebo (a sham or fake treatment). It is critical that phase III studies compare the new therapy or agent to the standard of care in order to determine actual benefit of a treatment. Phase III trials typically include hundreds to several thousand patients, and they often are of longer duration than earlier phase trials. Depending upon the disease, phase III trials can last anywhere from several months to several years. In the evaluation of drugs as a treatment for macular degeneration, most trials last a minimum of 1 year and typically 2 years. The large size and extended duration of phase III trials make them extremely expensive and complicated to run. Phase III trials are most likely to not only demonstrate the true treatment effects and benefits of a new treatment, but also the adverse events (side effects or complications).

Phase IV trials are referred to as postmarketing surveillance trials. They are designed to identify ongoing safety information and treatment benefits after a drug has permission from governing agencies, such as the FDA, to be sold. These trials may be mandated by the governing agency to continue to evaluate potential risks, or they may be initiated by the sponsor company to look for additional uses or marketing advantages. Phase IV studies may uncover less common adverse events that shorter, smaller phase III studies did not note. These trials often involve thousands of patients followed in a less rigorous manner but over a longer time period. Occasionally, side effects discovered in phase IV trials result in previously approved agents being no longer sold or restricted to limited use.

95. My doctor asked me to participate in a clinical trial. Why should I be a guinea pig?

Clinical trials are critical to advancing our ability to improve the care and treatment of many, if not most, diseases, including age-related macular degeneration. It was through clinical trials that the drug Lucentis was shown to be beneficial in the treatment of age-related macular degeneration. Lucentis was approved by the FDA in the summer of 2006; however, over 1000 patients were involved in the clinical trials years earlier and had the benefit of receiving this therapy years before the drug was approved. This instance does not mean that all clinical trials involve agents that will be beneficial in the treatment of age-related macular degeneration, but some may. Depending upon the state of your macular degeneration and the currently available treatment for the stage you are in, you may benefit from such trials. This important decision requires extensive and comprehensive discussions between you, your family, and your retina specialist. In addition, it may be beneficial to obtain a second opinion with regard to participation in the trial; however, the majority of trials are carefully designed and meticulously overseen, with the major emphasis being on patients' safety.

Nick's comment:

Personally, I was so pleased and grateful to be offered to participate in a trial. I would have done anything to be included. The alternative I had in front of me was going blind.

96. How do I know if a clinical trial is safe?

Clinical trials should be carefully designed and reviewed by at least two non-biased agencies. Typically, these include the FDA and an IRB (**institutional review board**). Clinical trials are usually designed under the guidance and consultation of leading experts in the field. Once the study design has been agreed upon, it is submitted to the FDA, whose experts review the study, both in terms of safety and in terms of potential benefit to patients. At the same time, the study is submitted to an IRB, whose emphasis is on patients' safety. Only after the study has received approval from both the FDA and the IRB is it offered to patients. Review by the FDA and IRB does not guarantee patients' safety or benefit. It does, however, ensure that experts in the field have reviewed the study and believe that the potential benefits to patients outweigh the potential risks.

Institutional review board

A committee formed to review and monitor human research to ensure patient safety and potential benefit.

Finally, in addition to review by the FDA and an IRB, many studies (and all phase III and larger phase II trials) have a data safety and monitoring committee, whose responsibility it is to review the study at regular intervals to ensure that no safety concerns have arisen.

Well-designed studies emphasize patients' safety as the number one priority. Patients considering clinical trials should discuss safety and potential benefit with their physician. Patients should be extremely careful and critical of studies that have not undergone the review process described here.

97. Are there natural therapies for treating age-related macular degeneration?

While numerous natural therapies are advertised for treating wet macular degeneration, there is no rigid clinical proof, such as that required by the FDA for treatments like Lucentis. Natural therapies, such as acupuncture, herbs, and other supplements or nutrients, have not been proven to impact wet macular degeneration. With regard to dry macular degeneration, eating a healthy diet with green leafy vegetables and vitamin supplementation as discussed in the AREDS questions (see Question 39) may help to prevent progression. Large randomized clinical trials (the types of trials that are most definitive for demonstrating the benefit or lack of benefit of a treatment) have not been performed for many of the nutritional supplements that are advertised in the press. This does not mean that these treatments are ineffective. It simply means that there is no definitive scientific evidence to support their use.

98. Can acupuncture help my macular degeneration?

Acupuncture is a treatment in which thin, long needles are inserted through the skin into various deep tissues of the body. Theoretically, it serves to correct imbalances in energy flow throughout the body. These imbalances may be of too great or too little flow. No randomized clinical trials have demonstrated the effi-

Acupuncture

A treatment in which thin, long needles are inserted through the skin into various deep tissues of the body in order to relieve pain or for other therapeutic purposes.

Other Treatments

105

cacy or safety of acupuncture for macular degeneration. Small series and anecdotal reports have reported benefits, but larger studies in which careful design and controls are critical have not been performed. As a result, the safety and benefit of acupuncture is not supported by the available scientific evidence.

99. What has genetic research revealed about macular degeneration?

There have been a number of recent breakthroughs with regard to genetics and macular degeneration. Researchers have known for years that macular degeneration ran in families and that patients with first-degree relatives with macular degeneration are several times more likely to develop the disease than those who do not have relatives with it. Several different researchers recently discovered a gene that encodes a variant of complement factor H, a protein that helps to regulate inflammation in the body. (Complement factor H, or CFH, plays an important role in the immune system, helping to regulate the body's response to infection.) The complement pathway is the body's way of responding to a variety of insults to the body, including viral and bacterial infections, cancer, and foreign materials. Several variants of genes encoding CFH have been discovered, some of which are protective and some of which confer increased risk of problems. CFH serves to shut down a person's immune response against infections from viruses or bacteria after the body has eliminated the infection. Patients with an abnormal variant of CFH are unable to accomplish this in the normal manner, leading to increased inflammation, a process that may play a role in the development of macular degeneration.

Other research has revealed variants of other genes involved in the complement pathway that also lead to defects in the body's inflammatory response and play a role in macular degeneration. Many of these genetic variants, when analyzed alone, have been associated with increased risk of developing macular degeneration, but when studied in combination the risk is often even greater. The discovery of genes associated with both wet and dry macular degeneration is leading to extensive research efforts in this direction. While it is still too early to know whether these breakthroughs will result in treatment advances, a genetic approach is certainly promising, as discussed in the final question. The possibilities for gene therapy are numerous. It is conceivable that patients could be tested years prior to the development of their disease, with prophylactic treatment initiated in those with the highest risk.

100. Will genetic testing help me to prevent macular degeneration from occurring or progressing, or allow me to get treated earlier?

At this time, genetic testing does not offer any advantages in terms of prevention of the onset of macular degeneration, prevention of progression of already existing disease, or earlier treatment of wet macular degeneration. This does not mean that it will not allow such options in the future. The recent discoveries of several variants of genes encoding for components of the complement system (the body's system that helps to clear pathogens such as viruses and bacteria from the body) has resulted in significant hope and excitement that ongoing research may ultimately allow clinicians to determine patients' risk, ideal therapy, and likelihood of treatment response based upon their genetic make-up. Others have hypothesized that at some point we may actually be able to study a patient's

The possibilities for gene therapy are numerous. It is conceivable that patients could be tested years prior to the development of their disease, with prophylactic treatment initiated in those with the highest risk.

Other Treatments

107

genetic code, and then modify their code in such a manner as to prevent the development of diseases such as macular degeneration before they ever occur. In addition, current research directed at dry macular degeneration and the prevention of wet macular degeneration from dry disease may offer the potential to utilize genetic analyses and offer such treatments to patients with certain genetic risk factors. However, these options are not available yet, and therefore genetic testing does not offer prevention or treatment benefits today. Risk modification, such as stopping smoking and eating a well-balanced diet with green leafy vegetables, is prudent in all patients, especially those with a strong family history of macular degeneration.

Glossary

Acupuncture: A treatment in which thin, long needles are inserted through the skin into various deep tissues of the body in order to relieve pain or for other therapeutic purposes.

Age-Related Eye Disease Study (AREDS): A multicenter national trial sponsored by the National Eye Institute, a branch of the National Institutes of Health, that showed that high levels of antioxidants and zinc (in combination with cupric oxide) reduced the risk of advanced macular degeneration and vision loss associated with this disease.

Amsler grid: A grid of vertical and horizontal straight lines in a square with a dot in the center designed as a screening test for detecting early macular abnormalities, such as wet macular degeneration.

Angiogenesis: The growth of new blood vessels. With respect to macular degeneration, this refers to the bad or pathologic growth of new blood vessels in wet macular degeneration.

Antiangiogenic agents: Drugs that prevent the growth of new blood vessels. Avastin and Lucentis are examples of such agents.

Antifibrotic: A drug or treatment that prevents or limits fibrosis (scarring).

Anti-inflammatory: A drug or treatment that prevents or inhibits inflammation.

Antioxidants: Substances that prevent oxidative damage in our body. For instance, spinach, collard greens, and kale are sources of antioxidants important in combating macular degeneration.

Anti-VEGF agents: Agents such as Lucentis and Avastin that block the growth of new blood vessels seen in wet macular degeneration by preventing VEGF from binding to its receptor in the eye. This prevents VEGF from stimulating the growth of new blood vessels. (VEGF is an abbreviation for vascular endothelial growth factor.)

Astigmatism: A condition in which abnormal shape of either a person's cornea or lens (or both) results in blurred vision.

Asymptomatic: Without symptoms.

Atrophy: A progressive breakdown or wasting away of a tissue, such as that seen in advanced dry macular degeneration.

Avastin: An anti-VEGF agent that is approved by the FDA for treatment of various cancers. Avastin's active component is similar to that of Lucentis. Avastin is used in the treatment of wet macular degeneration when administered by intravitreal injection. The use of Avastin for macular degeneration is considered off-label. Avastin is the commercial name for bevacizumab.

Betadine: A povidone-iodine scrub used prior to surgery or other form of medical treatment to disinfect the area to be treated.

Bevacizumab: The generic name for Avastin, an anti-VEGF agent that is approved by the FDA for treatment of various cancers. Bevacizumab has a similar active component to ranibizumab and is used in the treatment of wet macular degeneration when administered by intravitreal injection.

Bilberry: A dark, edible berry (similar to a blueberry) that has antioxidant activity.

Cataract: A clouding of one's natural lens.

CATT: Comparison of Age-Related Macular Degeneration Treatment Trial, a multicenter, randomized treatment trial evaluating the relative safety and efficacy of Lucentis versus Avastin.

Clinical trial: A study in humans that evaluates or compares new or established treatments in a specific predetermined manner (protocol).

Cold laser: A laser that works through the use of low power or intensity. With regard to macular degeneration, this refers to the use of photodynamic therapy, a laser that acts on abnormal vessels that have been activated by a photosensitizing dye (verteporfin).

Cornea: The clear, dome-shaped front part of the eye. The cornea helps to focus light onto the retina.

Cotton-wool spots: Small, fluffy white patches seen on retinal examination. They are secondary to ischemia and are often seen in diabetic retinopathy.

Diabetes mellitus: A disease in which abnormally high blood sugars lead to damage of various organs of the body, including the heart, kidneys, and eyes.

Diabetic retinopathy: Eye disease in which damage occurs secondary to high levels of blood sugar. Signs of diabetic retinopathy include retinal hemorrhages, cotton-wool spots, exudates, swelling, and new blood vessel growth.

Dilation: Enlargement of the pupils with eye drops.

Drusen: Yellow deposits beneath the retina, often indicative of macular degeneration. Drusen can be small and hard, large and soft, or anywhere in between. Large, soft drusen are associated with increased risk of developing more advanced stages of macular degeneration and vision loss. The singular form of drusen is druse.

Dry macular degeneration: The deterioration of the layers of the retina secondary to abnormal aging changes in the eye. This is the most common form of macular degeneration.

Exudative macular degeneration: Damage or breakdown of the retina secondary to a growth of abnormal blood vessels from beneath or in the retina. The abnormal blood vessels leak and bleed, resulting in vision loss.

Farsighted: An abnormality of the eye in which it cannot focus properly on near objects. This is often due to the eye being shorter than normal, or to the lens's inability to change shape appropriately.

Floaters: Spots of various size and shape within the eye, seen within a person's visual field. They may be inflammatory cells, pigment cells from tears in the retina, or small air bubbles from an intraocular injection.

Fluorescein angiogram (FA): A diagnostic test in which dye is injected into a patient's arm, and then photographed as it travels to and through the blood vessels of the retina. It helps retina specialists to detect abnormalities, such as new blood vessels in wet macular degeneration.

Geographic atrophy (GA): Geographic atrophy is the advanced form of dry macular degeneration in which

critical layers of the retina break down or degenerate entirely. When GA involves the center of the macula, severe vision loss may occur.

Glaucoma: A group of diseases that cause optic nerve damage and visual field loss as a result of intraocular pressure that is too high for the health of the eye. In some patients, this pressure is much higher than normal, but in others, even intraocular pressure that falls within the normal range may not be tolerated by an eye (so-called low-tension glaucoma). Glaucoma is typically treated with either eye drops or surgery (either intraocular or laser), or a combination of both.

Green leafy vegetables: Vegetables such as spinach, collard greens, and kale that are high in antioxidants. Lettuce is not high in such nutrients.

Hard drusen: Small, discrete, well-demarcated yellow deposits beneath the retina. Hard drusen are less likely to progress to more advanced stages of macular degeneration than soft drusen.

Histoplasmosis: A fungal infection that can occur in the retina. Its presence can lead to new blood vessel growth similar to that seen in wet macular degeneration.

Hyperpigmentation: Increased pigmentation (black or dark coloring) at the level of the retina. Hyperpigmentation indicates increased risk of macular degeneration progressing.

Indocyanine green (ICG): A dye test of the retina similar to fluorescein angiography but designed to evaluate the layer beneath the retina (the choroid). It is occasionally used to evaluate difficult or refractory cases of wet macular degeneration.

Institutional review board: A committee formed to review and monitor human research to ensure patient safety and potential benefit.

Intraretinal: Occurring within the retina, such as a hemorrhage or swelling.

Intravitreal: Into the vitreous cavity, the posterior compartment of the eye (which is occupied by a gel-like material called the vitreous). Lucentis and Avastin are injected into the vitreous cavity.

Legal blindness: Corrected vision (meaning with glasses if needed) that is 20/200 or worse in a patient's best-seeing eye.

Lid speculum: A piece of equipment that holds the eye open and the lids out of the way during procedures such as cataract surgery or intravitreal injections.

Low vision specialist: A trained eye care provider (typically an optometrist or ophthalmologist) who evaluates and manages patients with impaired vision. The specialist's goal is to maximize patients' visual deficit to allow them to perform their daily activities in the best manner possible despite their impairment.

Lucentis: An anti-VEGF treatment for wet age-related macular degeneration administered by injection. Lucentis is the commercial name for ranibizumab.

Lutein: An antioxidant found in green leafy vegetables that may be helpful in preventing or slowing macular degeneration.

Macugen: An approved anti-VEGF agent that is used in the treatment of wet macular degeneration.

Macula: The central area of the retina that is critical for fine, detailed vision.

Macular degeneration: The breakdown over time of the cells in the macula. Macular degeneration can occur from a number of causes, one of which is aging, and is referred to as age-related macular degeneration. Other causes of macular degeneration are poor nutrition and high myopia.

Nearsighted: An abnormality of the eye in which the eye cannot focus properly on distant objects. This is often due to the eye being longer than normal, or the cornea being too curved.

Omega-3 fatty acids: A family of unsaturated fatty acids that may have health benefits, including reducing heart disease and depression. Oily fish such as salmon and tuna are excellent sources of omega-3 fatty acids.

Ophthalmologist: A medical doctor trained in the medical and surgical management of eye diseases.

Optic nerve: The nerve that transmits impulses from the retina to the brain.

Optical coherence tomography (OCT): A noninvasive diagnostic imaging technique of the eye in which detailed cross-sectional images of the retina are obtained.

Optometrist: A licensed healthcare professional trained to provide primary eye care.

Pegaptanib: The generic name for Macugen, the first anti-VEGF treatment approved for the treatment of wet macular degeneration.

Periocular: Around the eye, but not in it. Periocular injections are outside the eye, unlike intravitreal injections, which are in the eye.

Photodynamic therapy: An approved therapy for wet macular degeneration in which a photosensitizing dye is injected into a patient's arm, and a cold or low-energy laser is used to treat the new blood vessels.

Ranibizumab: The generic name for Lucentis, an anti-VEGF treatment for wet age-related macular degeneration that is administered by intravitreal injection.

Refractive error: A focusing error of the eye that results in blurred vision. Hyperopia and myopia are examples of refractive errors.

Retina: The tissue lining the inner surface of the eye that receives light impulses and transmits them through the optic nerve to the brain.

Retinal pigment epithelium (RPE): The layer of cells beneath or outside the retina that serves to nourish the retinal photoreceptors (the light-sensing cells of the retina) as well as to remove or digest toxic byproducts generated in the photoreceptors.

Retina specialist: An ophthalmologist specially trained in the medical and/or surgical evaluation and management of diseases of the retina and vitreous.

Retinitis pigmentosa (RP): A group of inherited retinal disorders characterized by progressive visual field loss and difficulty with night vision.

Soft drusen: Poorly demarcated, amorphous yellow deposits beneath the retina. Soft drusen are more likely to progress to advanced stages of macular degeneration than hard drusen.

Steroids: Anti-inflammatory agents used to treat a variety of medical diseases. They may be administered systemically (intravenously or orally), by injection, or topically.

Strontium-90: A radioactive source used in the treatment of some cancers. It is also currently being studied in the treatment of wet macular degeneration.

Subconjunctival: Under the thin transparent covering of the white part of the eye.

Subretinal: Beneath the retina. Hemorrhages or fluid often accumulate beneath the retina in wet macular degeneration.

True blindness: Also called total blindness, the complete lack of sight. Patients aren't even able to see light.

Vascular endothelial growth factor (VEGF): A growth factor produced by various tissues in the body in response to various stimuli. In the eye, VEGF is a major factor involved in wet macular degeneration and stimulates the growth of new blood vessels seen in this disease.

Visual field: The total area in which vision exists while staring straight ahead at a fixed point. This typically refers to peripheral vision.

Wet macular degeneration: Damage and breakdown of the retina in which an abnormal growth of new blood vessels results in leakage and bleeding beneath and into the retina.

Zeaxanthin: A type of pigment located in the retina that has antioxidant properties.

Index

Index